CLINICAL
MANAGEMENT
OF DYSPHAGIA IN
ADULTS AND CHILDREN

Second Edition

THE REHABILITATION INSTITUTE OF CHICAGO PUBLICATION SERIES
Don A. Olson, PhD, Series Coordinator

Spinal Cord Injury: A Guide to Functional Outcomes in Physical Therapy Management

Lower Extremity Amputation: A Guide to Functional Outcomes in Physical Therapy Management, Second Edition

Stroke/Head Injury: A Guide to Functional Outcomes in Physical Therapy Management

Clinical Management of Right Hemisphere Dysfunction

Spinal Cord Injury: A Guide to Functional Outcomes in Occupational Therapy

Spinal Cord Injury: A Guide to Rehabilitation Nursing

Head Injury: A Guide to Functional Outcomes in Occupational Therapy Management

Speech/Language Treatment of the Aphasias: An Integrated Clinical Approach

Speech/Language Treatment of the Aphasias: Treatment Materials for Auditory Comprehension and Reading Comprehension

Speech/Language Treatment of the Aphasias: Treatment Materials for Oral Expression and Written Expression

Rehabilitation Nursing Procedures Manual

Psychological Management of Traumatic Brain Injuries in Children and Adolescents

Medical Management of Long-Term Disability

Psychological Aspects of Geriatric Rehabilitation

Clinical Management of Communication Problems in Adults with Traumatic Brain Injury

Cognition and Perception in the Stroke Patient: A Guide to Functional Outcomes in Occupational Therapy

Clinical Management of Dysphagia in Adults and Children

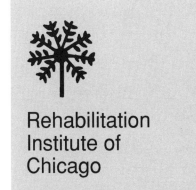

Rehabilitation
Institute of
Chicago

CLINICAL
MANAGEMENT
OF DYSPHAGIA IN
ADULTS AND CHILDREN

Second Edition

Leora Reiff Cherney, PhD., CCC-SLP

Clinical Researcher
Department of Communicative Disorders
Rehabilitation Institute of Chicago
Assistant Professor
Clinical Physical Medicine and Rehabilitation
Northwestern University Medical School
Chicago, Illinois

AN ASPEN PUBLICATION®
Aspen Publishers, Inc.
Gaithersburg, Maryland
1994

Library of Congress Cataloging in Publication Data

Cherney, Leora Reiff.
Clinical management of dysphagia in adults and children/ Leora Reiff
Cherney. -- 2nd ed.
p. cm. -- (Rehabilitation Institute of Chicago procedure
manual) (Rehabilitation Institute of Chicago publication series)
Rev. ed. of: Clinical evaluation of dysphagia. 1986.
Includes bibliographical references and index.
ISBN 0-8342-0376-6
1. Deglutition disorders--Handbooks, manuals, etc. 1. Cherney,
Leora Reiff.
Clinical evaluation of dysphagia. II. Title. III. Series.
IV. Series: Rehabilitation Institute of Chicago publication series.
[DNLM: 1. Deglutition Disorders. WI 250 C251c 1993]
RC815.2.C46 1993
617.5'31--dc20
DNLM/DLC
for Library of Congress
93-2073
CIP

The first edition of this work was published as *Clinical Evaluation of Dysphagia*.

The authors have made every effort to ensure the accuracy of the information herein, particularly
with regard to technique and procedure. However, appropriate information sources should be con-
sulted, especially for new or unfamiliar procedures. It is the responsibility of every practitioner to
evaluate the appropriateness of a particular opinion in the context of actual clinical situations and
with due consideration to new developments. Authors, editors, and the publisher cannot be held
responsible for any typographical or other errors found in this book.

Editorial Resources: Barbara Priest

Library of Congress Catalog Card Number: 93-2073

ISBN: 0-8342-0376-6

Printed in the United States of America

2   3   4   5

Table of Contents

Contributors

Maureen M. Boner, MS, CCC-SLP
Senior Speech-Language Pathologist
Alan J. Brown Center for Augmentative
   Communication Devices
Rehabilitation Institute of Chicago
Chicago, Illinois

Carol Addy Cantieri, MA, CCC-SLP
Speech-Language Pathologist
Waukesha Public Schools
Waukesha, Wisconsin

Leora Reiff Cherney, PhD, CCC-SLP
Clinical Researcher
Department of Communicative Disorders
Rehabilitation Institute of Chicago
Assistant Professor
Clinical Physical Medicine and Rehabilitation
Northwestern University Medical School
Chicago, Illinois

Anita S. Halper, MA, CCC-SLP
Director, Department of Communicative
   Disorders
Rehabilitation Institute of Chicago
Associate Professor
Clinical Physical Medicine and Rehabilitation
Northwestern University Medical School
Chicago, Illinois
Clinical Associate Professor
Department of Communication Sciences and
   Disorders
Northwestern University
Evanston, Illinois

Judy Michels Jelm, MS, CCC-SLP
Pediatric Speech and Language Services, Ltd.
Lisle, Illinois

Bonnie J.W. Martin, PhD, CCC-SLP
Program Director, Evelyn Trammell Voice
   and Swallowing Center
Clinical Manager, Communication and
   Swallowing Disorders
Saint Joseph's Hospital of Atlanta
Atlanta, Georgia
Adjunct Assistant Professor
University of Georgia
Athens, Georgia

Jean Jones Pannell, MA, CCC-SLP
Speech-Language Pathologist
Duxbury, Massachusetts

Wendy S. Perlin, MA, CCC-SLP
Senior Speech-Language Pathologist
Department of Communicative Disorders
Rehabilitation Institute of Chicago
Chicago, Illinois

Barbara C. Sonies, PhD, CCC-SLP
Chief, Speech-Language Pathology Section
Department of Rehabilitation Medicine
W. G. Magnuson Clinical Center
National Institutes of Health
Bethesda, Maryland

Series Preface

Over the past ten years, there has been increased involvement by the speech-language pathologist in the evaluation and treatment of dysphagia. As advances in medical technology have enabled people to survive increasingly more catastrophic illnesses and trauma, the numbers of individuals with dysphagia have increased significantly. We have been challenged to learn new techniques and specialized skills in order to effectively manage this problem. It is important for us as speech-language pathologists to continually expand our knowledge and experiences in this very important and potentially life-threatening area of treatment.

Rehabilitation medicine relies on an interdisciplinary approach to patient care. The way the treatment team works together, the approach they adopt and how they involve family members will determine the outcome of their treatment. This is essential in the management of dysphagia. However, it is usually the speech-language pathologist who designs and implements the feeding and swallowing program. This volume is intended to be a practical and useful guide to the clinician in the evaluation and treatment of adult and pediatric patients with dysphagia. It describes practical and functional approaches to maximizing the potential of these individuals. *Clinical Management of Dysphagia in Adults and Children* represents a major revision of the book *Clinical Evaluation of Dysphagia*, and has been expanded to include evaluation techniques for the pediatric population as well as treatment procedures for both children and adults.

This text is one in the series of Procedure Manuals that have been developed by the cooperative program between Aspen Publishers, Inc. and the Rehabilitation Institute of Chicago. It is our latest effort to share in an organized fashion our approaches to better management and care of our patients. The previous books for speech-language pathologists have focused on the management of patients with aphasia, right hemisphere dysfunction, and traumatic brain injury.

The contributors to this book are experienced clinicians with years of experience working with individuals with dysphagia. Their approaches are grounded on a scientific basis and have been used extensively in clinical practice. It is hoped that all speech-language pathologists working with dysphagic patients will find this book a helpful addition to their clinical libraries.

Anita S. Halper, M.A., CCC-SLP
Director of Communicative Disorders
Rehabilitation Institute of Chicago
Associate Professor
Clinical Physical Medicine and Rehabilitation
Northwestern University Medical School
Clinical Associate Professor
Department of Communication Sciences and Disorders
Northwestern University

Preface

According to the American Speech-Language-Hearing Association, an estimated 6 to 10 million Americans suffer some degree of dysphagia (Erlichman, 1989). Since the consequences of dysphagia may be serious and even life-threatening, a comprehensive, systematic, and careful approach to the management of swallowing disorders is essential.

The first step in the management of oropharyngeal dysphagia is the clinical examination. In 1986, *Clinical Evaluation of Dysphagia* was published as a guide to the administration and interpretation of the clinical examination, particularly in adults with neurogenic disorders. It included forms to aid in the documentation of the results of this examination, as well as a series of handouts for patient, family, and team education.

Since 1986, the American Speech-Language-Hearing Association has adopted position statements on the role of speech-language pathologists in providing services to dysphagic individuals (1986), and the knowledge and skills needed by speech-language pathologists who provide these services (1990). Changes in clinical practice have occurred including more widespread use of instrumental techniques, particularly videofluoroscopy, for evaluating dysphagia. In addition, the efficacy of intervention techniques for dysphagia has been recognized. At the same time, there has been an enormous increase in the amount of research on dysphagia.

With the generation of all this new information, there is a need for a practical text on dysphagia. *Clinical Management of Dysphagia in Adults and Children* has been expanded greatly from *Clinical Evaluation of Dysphagia*. In addition to chapters on dysphagia in both adults and children, the evaluation section includes a chapter on instrumental procedures. Chapters on treatment of dysphagia have also been added.

Clinical Management of Dysphagia in Adults and Children is divided into eight chapters. In Chapter 1, Cherney presents a summary of the neurophysiology of swallowing in adults and the changes in swallowing associated with aging and with a variety of common neurologic disorders. In Chapter 2, Boner and Perlin discuss the development of oral-motor and swallowing skills in the infant and child. They also summarize the feeding and swallowing problems that may accompany specific neurologic disorders in the pediatric population.

Chapters 3, 4, and 5 focus on the evaluation of dysphagia. In Chapter 3, Cherney, Pannell, and Cantieri provide guidelines for the clinical examination in adults, while Perlin and Boner discuss the clinical examination of dysphagia in infants and children in Chapter 4. Both chapters present a series of forms for documenting the results of the clinical examination. These forms were developed primarily to evaluate dysphagia in the neurologically impaired population, but they also may be used effectively to evaluate dysphagia associated with other etiologies. The forms may be reproduced for clinical use. Chapter 3 also includes handouts for patient, family, and team education, and an oral intake severity rating scale. In Chapter 5, Sonies presents a model for selecting appropriate instrumental techniques such as videofluoroscopy and ultrasonography for further differential diagnosis of dysphagia.

In Chapter 6, Martin relates dysphagia diagnosis to management in a discussion of indirect and direct approaches to treatment of adults. In Chapter 7, Jelm presents an overview of treatment approaches for children with dysphagia. Halper and Cherney, in Chapter 8, discuss the development of quality assurance monitors for dysphagia.

Dysphagia is a complex problem that requires an interdisciplinary team approach for effective management. All members of the dysphagia team would benefit from reading *Clinical Management of Dysphagia in Adults and Children*. The text is written primarily for the feeding specialist, however. The feeding specialist is typically a speech-language pathologist who has been specifically trained in the evaluation and treatment of oropharyngeal dysphagia (Erlichman, 1989).

Clinical Management of Dysphagia in Adults and Children will assist the clinician in gaining proficiency serving individuals with dysphagia. The up-to-date information and the systematic approach to evaluation and treatment should benefit both the clinician who is new to the field of dysphagia, and the more experienced clinician. It is hoped that this text will be helpful in daily clinical practice, and will be a welcome addition to your texts on dysphagia.

REFERENCES

American Speech-Language-Hearing Association, Ad Hoc Committee on Dysphagia. (1986). Ad Hoc Committee on Dysphagia Report. *ASHA, 29* (4), 57–58.

American Speech-Language-Hearing Association. (1990). Skills needed by speech-language pathologists providing services to dysphagic patients/clients. *ASHA, 32* (Suppl.2), 7–12.

Erlichman, M. (1989). Public health service assessment: The role of speech language pathologists in the management of dysphagia. Rockville, MD: National Center for Health Services Research and Health Care Technology Assessment.

Acknowledgments

I thank Maureen Boner, Senior Speech-Language Pathologist, Pamela Cole Carrico, Clinical Supervisor, and Wendy Perlin, Senior Speech-Language Pathologist, for their thoughtful comments on selected portions of the manuscript. A special note of thanks to Anita S. Halper, Director of the Department of Communicative Disorders, and Don A. Olson, Director of Education and Training, for their continued support of my professional endeavors.

♦ CHAPTER 1 ♦

Dysphagia in Adults with Neurologic Disorders: An Overview

Leora R. Cherney

PREVALENCE

Although swallowing difficulties have been described as components of several adult neurologic disorders, the exact prevalence of dysphagia in the adult neurologic population is neither widely documented nor agreed on in the literature. The prevalence differs depending on the types of institutions, the patients sampled, and the sampling methodology. For example, in an acute care setting, one-third of the patients may be dysphagic (Groher & Bukatman, 1986). The prevalence has been reported to increase to 42 percent in an acute rehabilitation facility (Pannell, Cantieri, & Cherney, 1984) and to approximately 60 percent in chronic care settings (Layne et al., 1989, Siebens et al., 1986). Several retrospective studies have reported that approximately one-quarter of patients with traumatic brain injury may be dysphagic (Cherney & Halper, 1989; Winstein, 1983), whereas one-third of patients with single hemispheric strokes may be dysphagic (Barer, 1989; Veis & Logemann, 1985; Young & Durant-Jones, 1990). In contrast to the retrospective studies, a prospective study by Gordon, Hewer and Wade (1987) indicated that as many as 42 percent of stroke patients may be dysphagic.

At the Rehabilitation Institute of Chicago (RIC), a retrospective study was conducted on 973 consecutive referrals between September 1990 and August 1991 to the Department of Communicative Disorders of adults with neurologic impairments. Of these, 307 patients (31.55 percent) presented with a dysphagia. At admission, the severity level for dysphagia in this patient sample ranged from severe to minimal, with most patients falling either in the severe range (31.6 percent) or in the mild-moderate range (29.32 percent). Severity levels were based on the functional oral intake scale, which is described in Chapter 3. Figures 1-1 and 1-2 illustrate these data.

Several etiologies have been attributed to dysphagia in the adults neurologic population. The most frequently occurring etiology in the RIC sample was stroke, which accounted for approximately half (153) of the 307 patients. Fifty-one patients (16.61 percent) presented with unilateral right hemisphere lesions, whereas 31 patients (10.1 percent) presented with unilateral left hemisphere lesions. Fifty-seven patients (18.57 percent) had bilateral cortical involvement. Fourteen patients (4.56 percent) had suffered a brain stem stroke.

The second most frequently occurring etiology was traumatic brain injury, which occurred in 60 patients (19.54 percent). Spinal cord injury and brain tumors each were present in 21 of the 307 patients (6.84 percent). Progressive neurologic disorders such as Parkinson's disease and multiple sclerosis occurred in 16 patients (5.21 percent). Thirty-six patients (11.73 percent) presented with a variety of other etiologies including

- postpolio syndrome
- encephalitis
- meningitis
- Guillain-Barré syndrome
- anoxia

Figure 1-3 displays the frequency of occurrence of each of the etiologies associated with dysphagia. Figure 1-4 compares the range of severity of dysphagia within each of the four most common groups:

- stroke
- traumatic brain injury
- spinal cord injury
- brain tumor

These data reflect the patient population of a large urban acute rehabilitation hospital and may not necessarily be indicative of other types of facilities. Nonetheless, they show that dysphagia frequently results from neurologic impairment and illustrate the variety of disorders that may be associated with dysphagia. Knowledge of the normal swallowing process is an essential first step in understanding these etiologies and their resultant dysphagias and in designing an effective management program for the patient with dysphagia.

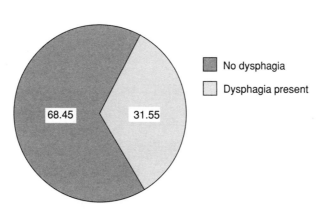

Figure 1-1 Prevalence of Dysphagia in 973 Adults with Neurologic Impairments Referred to the Communicative Disorders Department of an Acute Rehabilitation Hospital

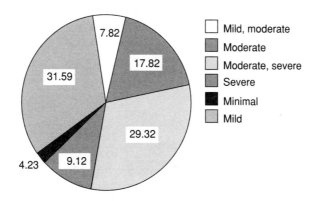

Figure 1-2 Range of Severity of Dysphagia in 307 Adults with Neurologic Impairment

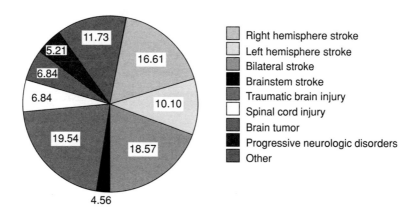

Figure 1-3 Etiologies Associated with Dysphagia in 307 Adults with Neurologic Impairment

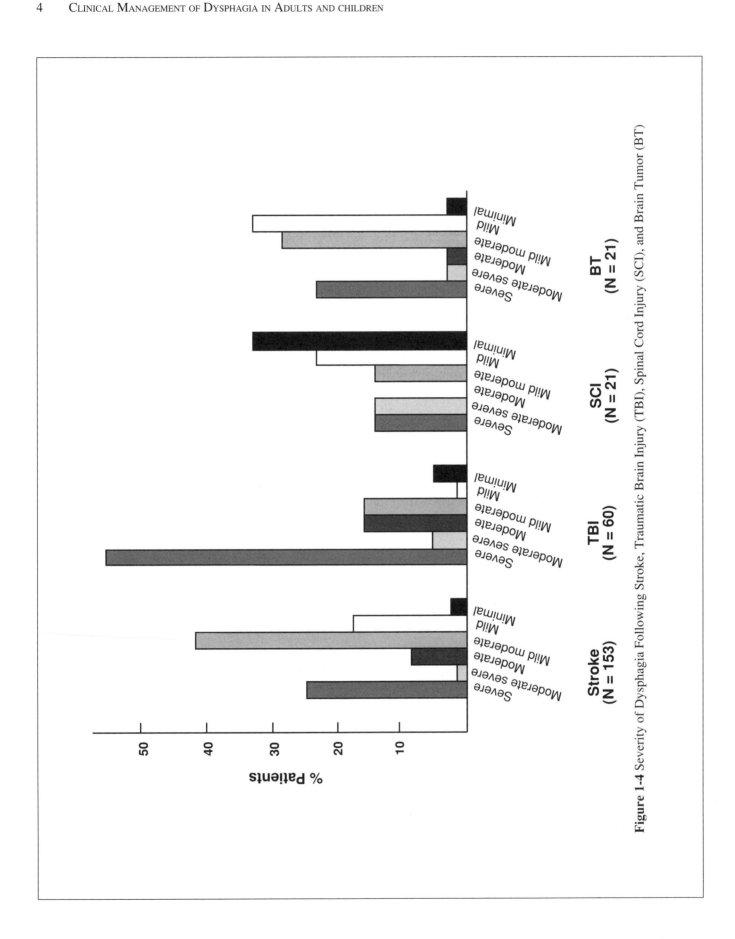

Figure 1-4 Severity of Dysphagia Following Stroke, Traumatic Brain Injury (TBI), Spinal Cord Injury (SCI), and Brain Tumor (BT)

NORMAL ORAL FEEDING

In normal oral feeding, the act of swallowing and the events that precede it typically involve a series of distinct stages. The anatomic structures and physiologic stages of normal swallowing are illustrated in Figures 1-5 to 1-7. Although most authorities generally agree on the sequence of events, there have been differences in opinion as to the number of stages into which the feeding process is divided and the terminology applied to each stage.

Anticipatory Phase

Leopold and Kagel (1983) coined this term to describe a stage of ingestion that occurs before any food reaches the mouth. During this stage, the decisions are made regarding type, rate, and quantity of oral intake.

Oral Phase

The oral phase of feeding has been divided into an oral "preparatory stage" (Leopold & Kagel, 1983; Logemann, 1983), during which time the food is manipulated and/or masticated, and an oral "transport stage" in which the tongue propels the food posteriorly. During the oral phase,

1. Labial seal is maintained to prevent food or liquid from leaking from the mouth.
2. Tension of the buccal musculature is maintained, to close off the lateral sulcus and prevent food particles from falling into the sulcus between the mandible and cheek (Logemann, 1983).
3. Depending on the consistency of the material, movement patterns of oral manipulation and mastication occur. The pattern of mastication involves rotary lateral movement of the mandible and tongue, which is repeated cyclically. Complex oral sensory input such as taste, touch, temperature, and proprioception help determine the oral activity required for appropriate bolus size and consistency (Doty, 1968).
4. Food particles are mixed with saliva and collected into a bolus that is held anteriorly and laterally by the tongue against the hard palate. The back of the tongue is usually elevated, with the soft palate pulled anteriorly against it to keep material in the oral cavity. During this preparatory stage, the airway is open, with the larynx and pharynx at rest. Nasal breathing may continue.
5. The tongue begins to propel food posteriorly. This is described as an anterior-to-posterior rolling action, with tongue elevation progressing sequentially more posteriorly to push the bolus backward (Logemann, 1983). It typically takes less than one second to complete.
6. The oral phase of the swallow is terminated when the bolus passes the anterior faucial arches, and the pharyngeal swallow is triggered.

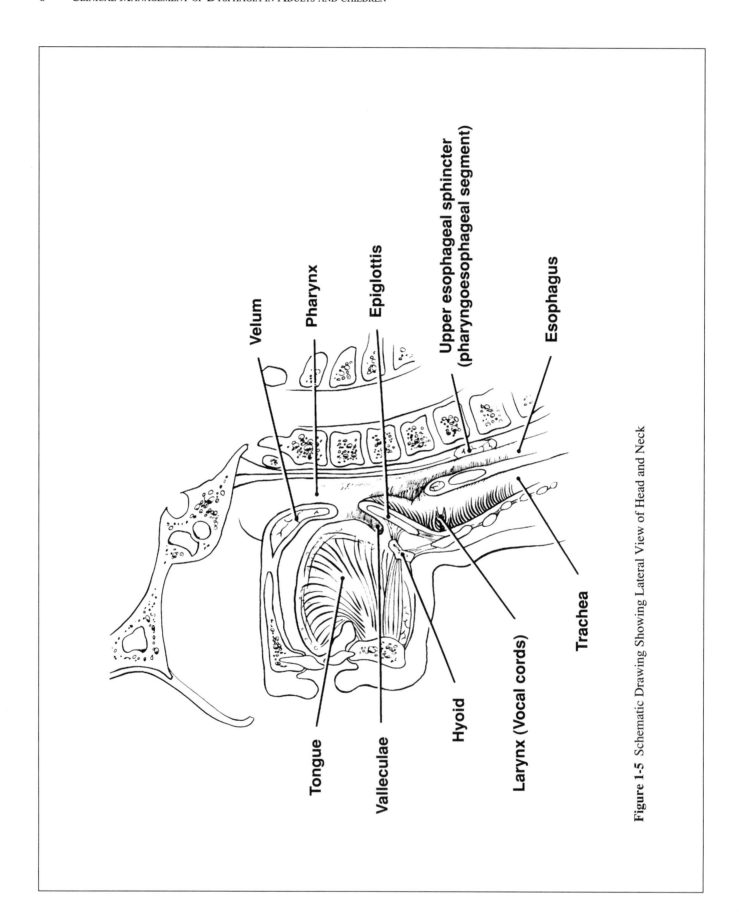

Figure 1-5 Schematic Drawing Showing Lateral View of Head and Neck

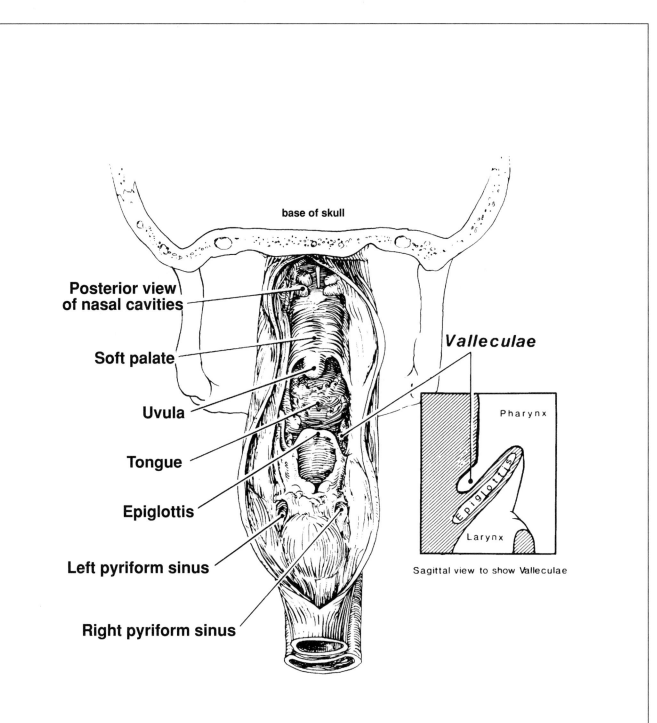

base of skull

Posterior view
of nasal cavities

Soft palate

Uvula

Tongue

Epiglottis

Left pyriform sinus

Right pyriform sinus

Valleculae

Pharynx

Epiglottis

Larynx

Sagittal view to show Valleculae

Figure 1-6 Schematic Drawing of Structures Anterior to Pharynx (Posterior View with Pharyngeal Constrictors Dissected Away)

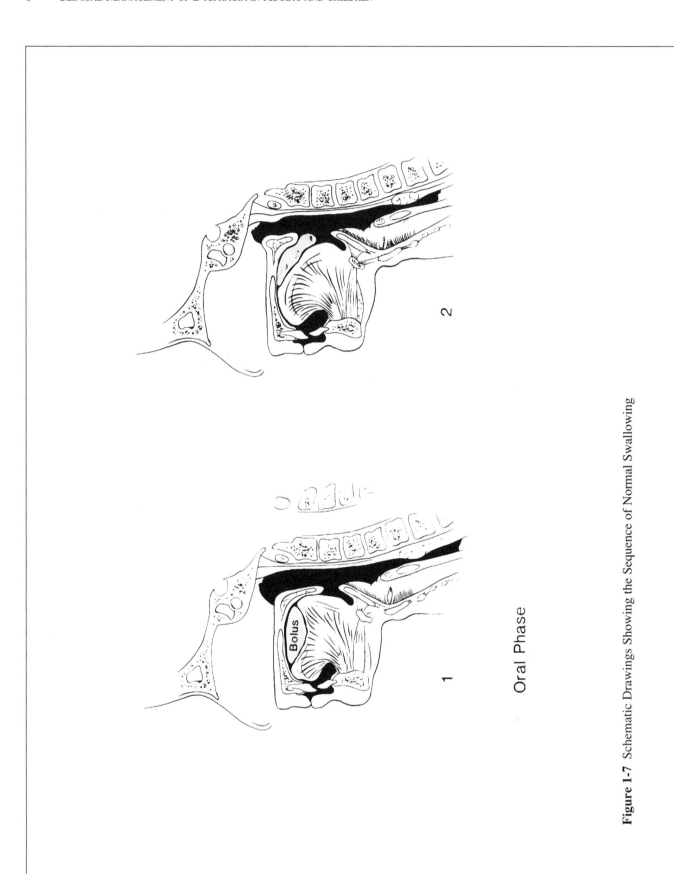

Oral Phase

Figure 1-7 Schematic Drawings Showing the Sequence of Normal Swallowing

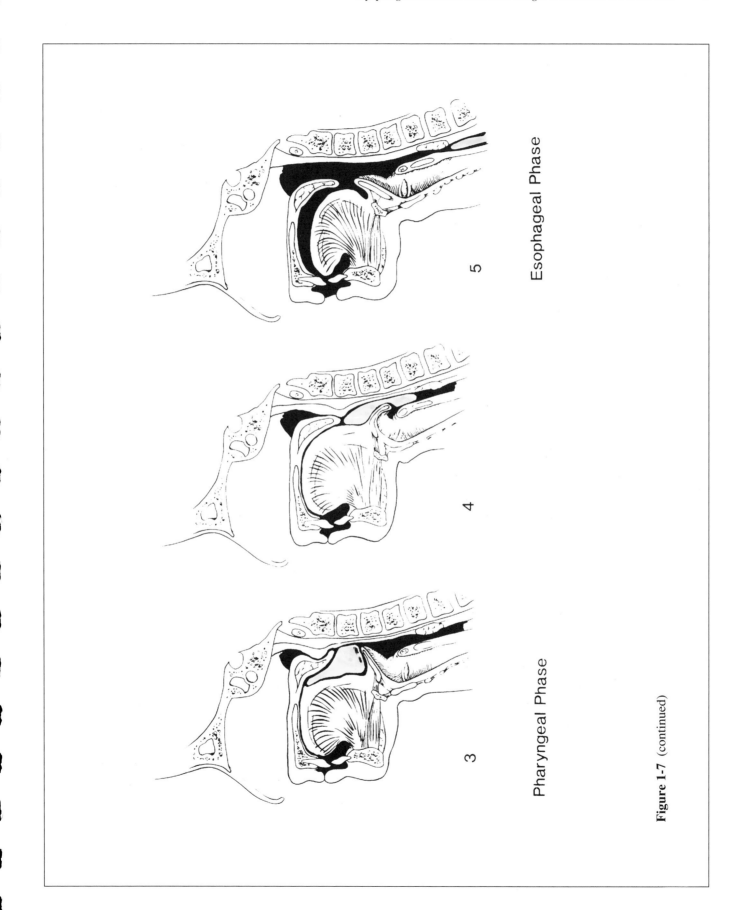

5

Esophageal Phase

4

3

Pharyngeal Phase

Figure 1-7 (continued)

The oral phase is under voluntary control. Sensory (afferent) information on taste and general sensation (pressure, light touch, pain, and temperature) are transmitted by cranial nerves V (trigeminal), VII (facial), and IX (glossopharyngeal) (Perlman, 1991). Motor (efferent) information is transmitted primarily by cranial nerves V, VII, and XII (hypoglossal) (Perlman, 1991). Mastication depends on the 5th cranial nerve. The muscles of the lips and cheeks depend primarily on the motor function of the 7th cranial nerve. The extrinsic and intrinsic muscles of the tongue are innervated mainly by the 12th (hypoglossal) cranial nerve.

Pharyngeal Phase

The pharyngeal phase begins with the triggering of the pharyngeal swallow. This causes several physiologic activities to occur simultaneously, the purpose of which is to control bolus propulsion and airway protection.

1. The tongue prevents reentry of food into the mouth, while the elevation and contraction of the velum results in complete closure of the velopharyngeal port to prevent material from entering the nasal cavity. This action is facilitated by contraction of the superior pharyngeal constrictor, which narrows the upper pharynx.

2. Initiation of pharyngeal peristalsis occurs. The bolus is carried by superior-to-inferior sequential muscular contractions of the superior, middle, and inferior pharyngeal constrictors into and through the pharynx to the cricopharyngeal sphincter. Movements of the tongue and larynx add to the pressures exerted on the bolus in the pharynx (Logemann, 1988). As the tongue retracts during the swallow, pressures are generated in the upper pharynx; as the larynx lowers at the end of the pharyngeal swallow, pressure is increased in the hypopharynx. Bolus transport through the pharynx typically takes less than 1 second (McConnell, Cerenko, Jackson, and Guffin, 1988).

3. Elevation, anterior displacement, and closure of the larynx occur to prevent material from entering the airway. Laryngeal closure begins at the level of the glottis (vocal folds), and progresses superiorly to the false cords and then to the epiglottis/aryepiglottic folds. Additional airway protection is provided by the epiglottis which descends and covers the laryngeal aditus, thereby diverting the bolus into the pyriform sinuses. Epiglottic movement results from the biomechanical effects of laryngeal elevation and anterior movement, bolus pressure from above, and tongue base retraction (Logemann, Kahrilas, Cheng, Pauloski, Gibbons, Rademaker, & Lin, 1992).

4. Relaxation of the cricopharyngeus, together with passive opening of the upper esophageal sphincter by laryngeal elevation and tilting (Kahrilas, Dodds, Dent, Logemann & Shaker, 1988) allows material to pass from the pharynx into the esophagus.

Multiple receptive sites for the elicitation of swallowing have been identified in the oropharyngeal region. However, the stimuli that trigger the pharyngeal swallow have not yet been clearly defined. Besides the presence of the bolus, the action of the tongue as it propels the bolus posteriorly may stimulate receptors in the oropharyngeal region to trigger the pharyngeal swallow (Logemann, 1988). The sensory receptors in the oropharynx connect primarily with the 9th and 10th cranial nerves, which transmit signals to the paired "swallowing centers" in the reticular formation of the medulla within the brain stem (Miller, 1986). Here, a pattern recognition system has been hypothesized. The incoming stimuli are identified as appropriate for a swallow, and the required preprogrammed neuromuscular response is generated, with motor impulses being sent to the controlling nuclei and the axons of the 9th, 10th, and 12th cranial nerves. Also, descending cortical input may modify the threshold of reflexively evoked swallowing and may be important pathways in the voluntary elicitation of swallowing (Miller, 1986).

Esophageal Phase

The esophageal phase commences with the lowering of the larynx, the contraction of the cricopharyngeus muscle to guard against regurgitation of food particles into the respiratory system, and the resumption of respiration. Together with gravity, a complex series of peristaltic waves transports the bolus through the esophagus and into the stomach. This takes an average time of 8 seconds (Miller, 1982).

AGE-RELATED CHANGES IN SWALLOWING

Any discussion of the physiology of swallowing should consider the effects of aging on the swallowing process. Research seems to indicate that in the healthy elderly person, age-related changes are subtle; they may slow the swallowing process, but they do not interfere greatly with everyday feeding skills (Ekberg & Feinberg, 1991; Robbins et al., 1992; Sonies, Parent, Morrish, & Baum, 1988; Tracy et al., 1989b). Sonies (1992a) described these age-related changes as subclinical; they are not considered to be a "disorder" because the effects on the swallowing process are negligible and usually only detected in controlled investigations. Furthermore, because the age-related changes are insidious and gradual, the older healthy individual can easily adjust to them. For example, difficult consistencies of food may be avoided, the size of the bolus may be reduced, or food may be chewed more thoroughly (Sonies, 1992a).

Rather than age per se, the general health status of the individual may determine the presence and severity of a swallowing problem. In the frail aged individual, decreased physical conditioning and reduced cognitive skills may interact with the age-related changes. Often the individual is unable to make the necessary adaptations and compensations that the healthy individual does. Chewing and swallowing difficulties that interfere with functional feeding and with the ability to maintain adequate nutrition may result. Furthermore, swallowing may be affected by changes that are secondary to other systemic conditions or are the result of pharmacologic intervention for other disorders.

Table 1-1 reviews the age-related changes in healthy individuals that occur for each stage of the swallowing process and then compares them with the changes typical of the frail aged individual. These changes can be compared and contrasted with the swallowing problems associated with neurologic impairment, as listed in Table 1-2.

DISTURBANCES IN ORAL FEEDING

The oral feeding process, as outlined above, is dependent on a highly coordinated and integrated sequence of stages, which may be interrupted at any one or more points. Specific anatomic and neuromuscular disorders may result in aspiration, whereby food particles penetrate the larynx and enter the airway below the true vocal folds. Aspiration may occur before, during, or after the initiation of the pharyngeal swallow. The presence of aspiration is clinically significant, because of the possible development of pulmonary complications, including aspiration pneumonia (Langmore, 1991).

Table 1-2 lists some of the typical problems and their effects that result from neurologic damage in the adult with dysphagia (Logemann, 1983, 1988). The problems usually occur in different combinations, depending on the specific patient and the nature of the disease. The different neurologic diseases that may cause dysphagia are discussed in the following section.

Table 1-1 Swallowing Problems in the Healthy and Frail Aged Adult

	Healthy Aged	*Frail Aged*
Anticipatory Stage (Logemann, 1990)	No significant alterations	Cognitive deficits (e.g., attention, memory) may compound the neuromuscular changes of normal aging and interfere with the spontaneous use of compensatory techniques
		Depression may cause poor food intake and weight loss
Oral Stage (Ekberg & Feinberg, 1991; Hughes et al., 1987; Sonies et al., 1988)		Reduced endurance may interfere with oral-motor function and result in slow eating and decreased food intake

continues

Table 1-1 continued

	Healthy Aged	*Frail Aged*
Oral Stage (continued) (Ekberg & Feinberg, 1991; Hughes et al., 1987; Sonies et al., 1988)	Loss of muscle tone and atrophy of lips and tongue may result in slower manipulation of food. Pattern of multiple lingual gestures may be present	Reduced labial closure and reduced oral sensitivity may result in drooling Reduced lingual strength, range, rate, and sensation may result in reduced lingual manipulation and propulsion of the bolus
	Tooth loss may result in increased time and effort for chewing	Tooth loss and mandibular weakness or temporomandibular joint dislocation may result in reduced mastication
	Reduced sensitivity to taste may result in decreased appetite	Xerostomia or reduced salivation may interfere with bolus formation and propulsion. Associated oral soreness and ulceration may discourage feeding and result in decreased nutritional status
Pharyngeal Stage (Ekberg & Feinberg, 1991; Robbins et al., 1992; Tracy et al., 1989b)	Only minimal alterations in transit time. However, the following subtle changes may occur: • increased delay of the pharyngeal swallow • increased duration of the pharyngeal swallow response • decreased peristaltic amplitude and velocity • increased maximal laryngeal elevation • slower descent of the larynx • decreased duration of upper esophageal sphincter opening	Increased transit time
Esophageal Stage (Ekberg & Feinberg, 1991; Sheth & Diner, 1988)	No clinically significant alterations, although decreased amplitude of esophageal peristalsis may occur	Increased transit time Gastroesophageal reflux

Source: Adapted from "Speech and swallowing disorders" by L.R. Cherney, in *Geriatric Medicine,* J.E. Morley (Ed.), in press. Reprinted by permission.

Table 1-2 Dysphagic Problems Related to Neurologic Damage

Oral Phase

Problem	Effect
Reduced labial closure	Food or liquid may leak from the mouth
Reduced lateral and vertical range of tongue movement	Reduced ability to manipulate food in the mouth during mastication, to form and hold the bolus, and to propel the food posteriorly. This results in separation of food throughout the oral cavity; particles may fall over the base of the tongue into the pharynx and be partially aspirated *before* the initiation of the pharyngeal swallow
Reduced buccal tension	Food may fall into the lateral sulcus during mastication and may be difficult to retrieve
Reduced oral sensitivity	Material that lodges in areas of reduced sensitivity may not be felt; food particles may fall over the base of the tongue and be aspirated *before* the initiation of the pharyngeal swallow

Pharyngeal Phase

Problem	Effect
Delayed/absent pharyngeal swallow	Pooling in the valleculae or pyriform sinuses may occur, with overflow into the airway and aspiration *before* the pharyngeal swallow is initiated
Inadequate velopharyngeal closure	Material may enter the nasal cavity, resulting in possible nasal regurgitation

continues

Table 1-2 continued

Problem	Effect
Reduced laryngeal closure	Airway protection is compromised with aspiration occurring *during* the swallow
Reduced pharyngeal peristalsis	Residue may remain in the valleculae and pyriform sinuses; if particles fall into the airway, aspiration may occur *after* the pharyngeal swallow
Reduced laryngeal elevation	Some material may remain on top of the larynx; aspiration may occur *after* the swallow when the larynx opens to restore respiration
Upper esophageal sphincter dysfunction	If the cricopharyngeus does not relax, or if the sphincter opens too late or closes too soon, material may collect in the pyriform sinuses, with overflow into the airway, and aspiration evident *after* the swallow

Esophageal Phase

Problem	Effect
Lax cricopharyngeus	A bolus of material that has entered the esophagus may reflux back into the pharynx and spill into the airway, causing aspiration *after* the swallow
Reduced peristalsis	Material may remain in the esophagus because of reduced movement of the bolus

COMMON NEUROLOGIC DISORDERS ASSOCIATED WITH DYSPHAGIA

This section lists the more common disorders that are associated with feeding and swallowing problems and summarizes the symptoms of dysphagia that frequently occur in each disorder. This section is not intended to be all inclusive but rather serves to highlight the predominant characteristics of each disorder. Patients may not present with all the feeding and swallowing problems highlighted, or they may present with additional symptoms. Although patients may have similar disorders, their swallowing problems may differ clinically. For more detailed information about a specific disorder, it is suggested that the reader refer to the many recent sources cited.

Vascular Disease

Swallowing problems frequently occur after stroke (Barer, 1989; Gordon et al., 1987; Gresham, 1990). The specific symptoms vary according to the site and size of the lesion (i.e., cortical versus brain stem; left versus right; anterior versus posterior; unilateral versus bilateral). For instance, dysphagia is more commonly associated with more anterior lesions (Logemann, 1983; Meadows, 1973). Hemispheric infarcts involving larger vascular territories (i.e., middle cerebral artery, posterior cerebral artery) tend to have a higher incidence of aspiration than small-territory hemispheric infarcts (Alberts, Horner, Gray, & Brazer, 1992).

Cortical Stroke

Robbins and Levine (1988) found that left cortical stroke was characterized mainly by impaired oral stage function, whereas right cortical stroke was associated primarily with pharyngeal stasis, laryngeal penetration, and aspiration. In contrast, other researchers found that most of their cortical stroke patients experienced difficulty in both the oral and pharyngeal phases of swallowing, regardless of anatomic location of the stroke (Chen, Ott, Peele, & Gelfand, 1990). Johnson, McKenzie, Rosenquist, Lieberman, and Sievers (1992) found no difference in pharyngeal transit times for left- and right-sided lesions. Furthermore, Alberts et al., (1992) suggested that there is no association between stroke location and the occurrence of aspiration. Because the research findings are conflicting, it is essential that each individual patient be evaluated carefully so that their specific swallowing symptoms can be identified.

The symptoms of swallowing disorders listed below may occur in isolation, or more commonly, in clusters of two or more symptoms (Gresham, 1990; Veis & Logemann, 1985).

With left (dominant) hemisphere involvement, the following may be observed (Chen et al., 1990; Robbins & Levine, 1988; Veis & Logemann, 1985):

- contralateral reductions in labial, lingual, and mandibular strength, rate, range of motion, and sensation

- delayed pharyngeal swallow
- contralateral reductions in pharyngeal peristalsis

With right (nondominant) hemisphere involvement the following symptoms may be observed (Chen et al., 1990; Logemann, 1990; Leopold & Kagel, 1983; Miller & Groher, 1982; Robbins & Levine, 1988; Veis & Logemann, 1985; Wyse, Grant, & Redenbaugh, 1984):

- contralateral reductions in labial, lingual, and mandibular strength, rate, range of motion, and sensation
- delayed pharyngeal swallow
- contralateral reductions in pharyngeal peristalsis
- reduced orientation, perceptual deficits, attention deficits, impulsivity, errors in judgment, and loss of intellectual control over swallowing, compounding the neuromuscular symptoms and making use of compensatory techniques difficult

With bilateral hemisphere involvement, the following symptoms may be observed (Celifarco, Gerard, Faegenburg, & Burakoff, 1990; Hellemans, Pelemans, & Van Trappen, 1981; Horner, Massey, & Brazer, 1990; Veis & Logemann, 1985):

- reduced labial, lingual, and mandibular strength, rate, range of motion, and sensation
- delayed pharyngeal swallow
- reduced pharyngeal peristalsis
- incomplete laryngeal elevation and closure
- upper esophageal sphincter involvement

Brain Stem Stroke

Brain stem stroke may result in these symptoms (Donner, 1974; Hellemans et al., 1981; Horner, Buoyer, Alberts, & Helms, 1991; Veis & Logemann, 1985):

- reduced labial, lingual, and mandibular strength, rate, range of motion, and sensation
- absent or delayed initiation of the pharyngeal swallow
- reduced pharyngeal peristalsis
- reduced laryngeal adduction
- upper esophageal sphincter involvement

Traumatic Brain Injury

Symptoms vary according to the location and extent of the head injury. Also, the interaction of cognitive, behavioral, and linguistic impairments with the dysphagia must be considered. The following symptoms have been described in patients with traumatic brain injury (Cherney & Halper, 1989; Field & Weiss, 1989; Lazarus & Logemann, 1987; Logemann, 1990; Tippett, Palmer, & Linden, 1987; Winstein, 1983):

- cognitive problems including attentional deficits, impulsivity, orientation problems, memory deficits, reduced organization, and poor reasoning and judgment
- reduced tongue control
- prolonged oral transit
- delayed or absent pharyngeal swallow
- reduced pharyngeal peristalsis
- laryngeal penetration, often without a cough reflex
- tracheoesophageal fistula, often as a result of long-term intubation

Spinal Cord Injury

The following symptoms have been described in patients with cervical spinal cord injury (Lazzara, Lazarus, & Logemann, 1985; Tracy, Logemann, & Kahrilas, 1989a; Veis & Logemann, 1991):

- absent or delayed pharyngeal swallow
- reduced pharyngeal peristalsis
- reduced base of tongue retraction (resulting in residue in the valleculae)
- reduced laryngeal elevation and/or closure
- upper esophageal sphincter dysfunction (reduced width and duration of upper esophageal sphincter opening)

The specific swallowing symptoms and the severity of the dysphagia may vary depending on the level of the injury (Lazzara et al., 1985). Although Veis and Logemann (1991) did not find a relationship between swallowing problems and either the effects of cervical spine stabilization (surgical fusion and bracing) or the respiratory status (tracheostomy or mechanical ventilation) of the patient, these factors should be considered when evaluating and treating dysphagia in spinal cord–injured patients.

Tumors

Central nervous system tumors may be cortical, subcortical, unilateral, bilateral, diffuse, or confined to a specific lobe of the brain (Sonies, 1987). Specific feeding and swallowing symptoms will depend on their location and size.

Cranial nerve tumors will affect swallowing if they involve any of the nerves that control oral-pharyngeal-laryngeal function. These are the trigeminal (V), facial (VII), glossopharyngeal (IX), vagus (X), spinal accessory (XI), and hypoglossal (XII) cranial nerves.

The effects of neurosurgery, chemotherapy, and/or radiation therapy on swallowing should also be considered.

Multiple Sclerosis

Multiple sclerosis is associated with multiple lesions involving demyelination of the cortex, cerebellum, brain stem, and spinal cord. It presents a fluctuating pattern of remission and exacerbation or one of gradual progression (Darley, Aronson, & Brown, 1975). The following symptoms may be observed (Daly, Code, & Anderson, 1962; Hellemans et al., 1981; Herrera et al., 1990; Logemann, 1983; Silbiger, Pikielney, & Donner, 1967):

- impaired ability to hold the bolus anteriorly and laterally
- delayed initiation of the pharyngeal swallow
- reduced pharyngeal peristalsis
- laryngeal adduction (later stages of the disease)

Amyotrophic Lateral Sclerosis

In this form of motor neuron disease, both upper and lower motor neurons are affected, resulting in a mixture of spasticity and flaccid muscular weakness and atrophy. The specific swallowing symptoms depend on the course of the disease and the particular motor neurons affected. The following symptoms may be observed (Bosma & Brodie, 1969; Carpenter, McDonald, & Howard, 1978; Dworkin & Hartman, 1979; Fischer, Ellison, Thayer, Spiro, & Glaser, 1965; Hillel & Miller, 1989; Logemann, 1983; Robbins, 1987):

- difficulty with lingual control and oral manipulation of bolus
- nasal regurgitation
- delayed initiation of the pharyngeal swallow
- reduced pharyngeal peristalsis
- reduced laryngeal elevation as the disease progresses
- upper esophageal sphincter dysfunction
- esophageal reflux
- esophageal dysmotility
- progressive respiratory insufficiency and weakness of abdominal muscles

Progressive Neurologic Diseases: Movement Disorders

Parkinsonism

Parkinsonism is associated with degeneration of pigmented neurons in the substantia nigra and is characterized by tremor, rigidity, and bradykinesia. Dysphagia is a frequent and potentially serious complication of Parkinson's disease. The following symptoms may be observed (Bushman, Dobmeyer, Leeker, & Perlmutter, 1989; Calne, Shaw, Spiers, & Stern, 1970; Eadie & Tyrer, 1965; Hellemans et al., 1981; Lieberman et al., 1980; Logemann, Blonsky, & Boshes, 1975; Nowack, Hatelid, & Sohn, 1977; Palmer, 1974; Robbins, Logemann, & Kirshner, 1986; Silbiger et al., 1967; Stroudley & Walsh, 1991):

- tongue tremor with reduced initiation of lingual movement
- repetitive tongue-pumping action
- lingual festination (posterior part of tongue remains elevated, preventing passage of bolus into the pharynx)
- delayed pharyngeal swallow
- reduced pharyngeal peristalsis
- inadequate laryngeal elevation and/or closure
- laryngeal penetration, often with absence of coughing
- repetitive, involuntary reflux from the valleculae and pyriform sinuses into the oral cavity
- upper esophageal sphincter dysfunction
- reduced esophageal peristalsis

Progressive Supranuclear Palsy

In progressive supranuclear palsy, basal ganglia, and structures of the cerebellum and brain stem are affected. This progressive disease is characterized by opthalmoplegia of vertical gaze, pseudobulbar palsy, dysarthria, dystonia, and severe rigidity of the head and neck producing a backward retracted head position (Klawans & Tanner, 1984). The following feeding and swallowing symptoms may be observed (Sonies, 1992b):

- hyperextended neck posture
- excessive lingual and velar movements
- impaired oral anterior–posterior bolus transport
- delayed initiation of the pharyngeal swallow

Huntington's Disease

Huntington's disease is a hereditary neurodegenerative disease of the central nervous system characterized by involuntary movements, dementia, and emotional impairment. The swallowing problems listed below are typical of Huntington's chorea (Kagel & Leopold, 1992; Leopold & Kagel, 1975; Miller & Groher, 1992; Morrell, 1992; Silbiger et al., 1967):

- neck and trunk hyperextension
- involuntary movement of body, head, and oral motor structures that interfere with oral phase
- absent or inefficient mastication
- irregular breathing patterns that interrupt the normal reciprocal respiration–deglutition cycle (inspiration during the swallow may result in aspiration)
- pharyngeal dysmotility
- uncoordinated and asynchronous vocal cord adduction/abduction

However, a small percentage of patients also present with varying degrees of bradykinesia and rigidity. In these patients, the dysphagia may include symptoms similar to those of Parkinson's disease (Kagel & Leopold, 1992).

Disorders of the Neuromuscular Junction and Muscle

Muscular Dystrophy

Myotonic Dystrophy. Myotonic dystrophy is characterized by myotonia followed by muscle atrophy, especially to muscles of the face and neck. The following symptoms may be observed (Casey & Aminoff, 1971; Hellemans et al., 1981; Ludman, 1962; Pierce, Creamer, & MacDermot, 1965):

- generalized pharyngeal weakness
- cricopharyngeal dysfunction: prolonged contraction and/or relaxation
- reduced esophageal peristalsis

Oculopharyngeal Muscular Dystrophy. Oculopharyngeal muscular dystrophy is a chronic, progressive myogenic disorder occurring in older age groups and affecting ocular and pharyngeal muscles. The following symptoms may be observed (Duranceau, Leterdre, Clemont, Levesque, & Barbeau, 1978; Hellemans et al., 1981; Logemann, 1983; Silbiger et al., 1967:

- reduced pharyngeal peristalsis
- upper esophageal sphincter dysfunction

Myasthenia Gravis

Myasthenia Gravis is an autoimmune disorder characterized by fatigue and exhaustion of the muscular system caused by impaired conduction at the myoneural junction. The following symptoms may be observed (Donner, 1974; Fischer et al., 1965; Hellemans et al., 1981; Murray, 1962; Silbiger et al., 1967):

- overall reduction in oral preparatory phase
- reduced lingual motility
- nasal regurgitation
- reduced pharyngeal peristalsis
- slowed esophageal transit

Because of the tendency for the musculature to fatigue easily, symptoms become more obvious on repeated swallowing attempts. Chewing and swallowing deteriorate toward the end of a meal and toward the end of the day.

Infection

Postpolio Syndrome

This syndrome refers to symptoms experienced by survivors of the poliomyelitis virus infection. The symptoms include fatigue, pain in muscles and/or joints, and muscle weakness. The symptoms usually begin several decades after recovery from the acute illness and may be progressive. Swallowing problems have been described in postpolio individuals. The most common characteristics of their dysphagia are as follows (Bucholz & Jones, 1991; Coelho & Ferranti, 1988; 1991; Jones, Buchholz, Ravich, & Donner, 1992; Silbergleit, Waring, Sullivan, & Maynard, 1991; Sonies & Dalakas, 1991):

- excessive tongue pumping and lingual movements
- difficulty with bolus control because of lingual and/or velar weakness
- delayed pharyngeal swallow
- reduced pharyngeal peristalsis (transit), often asymmetric
- laryngeal penetration, often with absence of coughing
- upper esophageal sphincter dysfunction
- gastroesophageal reflux and disordered esophageal motility

Acquired Immune Deficiency Syndrome

Acquired immune deficiency syndrome (AIDS) may compromise swallowing function as a result of

- central nervous system complications of human immunodeficiency virus (HIV)
- local infection and neoplasms involving the mouth, pharynx, larynx, esophagus, and lungs (Groher, 1991)

HIV-related central nervous system syndromes include HIV encephalitis, cryptococcal meningitis, progressive multifocal leukoencephalopathy, and central nervous system lymphoma (Singer, 1991). The specific nature of the swallowing impairment coincides with the site of involvement (Groher, 1991).

Candidiasis (thrush) is a fungal infection that commonly causes odonophagia (painful swallowing) and dysphagia in patients with AIDS (Raufman, 1988). The lesions appear as soft white, slightly elevated plaques on the tongue or on the oral, pharyngeal, or esophageal mucosa. Kaposi's sarcoma also may cause odonophagia in patients with AIDS. This fungal inflammation may be found in any part of the oral mucosa but most commonly on the hard palate (Greenspan & Greenspan, 1988). Odonophagia may be one of the first symptoms of acute HIV infection (Rabeneck et al., 1990).

Dementia

Dementia is an acquired progressive deterioration of intellectual function caused by changes in the central nervous system. A constellation of behavioral abnormalities is evident, with compromise in several spheres of mental activity including cognition, language, memory, visuospatial skills, emotion, and personality (Cummings & Benson, 1983). Dementia may be caused by several different pathologies, the most common being Alzheimer's disease. Multi-infarct dementia results from multiple small vascular lesions. Other disorders associated with dementia include

- Parkinson's disease
- multiple sclerosis
- Huntington's disease
- Pick's disease
- Creutzfeldt-Jakob disease

The following feeding and swallowing problems may be present in dementia (Cherney, in press; Feinberg & Ekberg, 1991; Logemann, 1990):

- cognitive deficits (e.g., reduced attention, orientation, memory, perception, and judgment) may compound the neuromuscular changes of normal aging and interfere with the spontaneous use of compensatory techniques
- reduced initiation of oral preparatory lingual and mandibular movements
- protracted or nonpurposeful bolus processing
- loss of bolus control
- prolonged oral transit
- delayed pharyngeal swallow

Oncologic Conditions Affecting Swallowing

Although this is not a direct result of a neurologic problem, the feeding specialist should be aware of the effects of oncologic conditions on swallowing.

Dysphagia may result after surgical treatment for oral, pharyngeal, and laryngeal cancer. The resultant swallowing deficits will depend on the amount of ablative surgery, the degree of reconstructive surgery, the presence of scar tissue, and the integrity of the remaining oropharyngeal and laryngeal structures (Groher & Gonzalez, 1992; Logemann, 1985). For example, patients with resections of the tongue, floor of the mouth, and mandible may experience difficulty with mastication, bolus control, and anteroposterior propulsion. A pharyngeal resection may result in a reduction in peristalsis, with residual food left in the pharynx after the swallow. After a hemilaryngectomy, the ability to close the airway tightly enough to prevent aspiration of liquids is diminished. After a total laryngectomy, there are often changes in structure that may affect swallowing, including upper esophageal sphincter dysfunction.

Swallowing also may be compromised by the potential side effects of pre- and post-operative irradiation. These may include (Groher & Gonzalez, 1992)

- oral and pharyngeal inflammation with subsequent pain in the soft tissues and bone
- changes in salivary flow (decreased volume and/or thicker consistency)
- loss of taste and appetite

The patient who complains of any new swallowing problem should be referred back to the surgeon because changes in swallowing may be a symptom of recurrence of the disease (Logemann, 1985).

SUMMARY

This chapter has reviewed the physiology of swallowing, described changes in swallowing that occur with advancing age, and identified several neurologic disorders that are associated with dysphagia. This information is important for the clinician who evaluates and treats dysphagia in adults with neurologic impairments.

REFERENCES

Alberts, M.J., Horner, J., Gray, L., & Brazer, S.R. (1992). Aspiration after stroke: Lesion analysis by brain MRI. *Dysphagia, 7,* 170–173.

Barer, D.H. (1989). The natural history and functional consequences of dysphagia after hemispheric stroke. *Journal of Neurology, Neurosurgery, and Psychiatry, 52,* 236–241.

Bosma, J.F., & Brodie, D.R. (1969). Disabilities of the pharynx in ALS as demonstrated by cineradiography. *Radiology, 92,* 97-103.

Buchholz, D., & Jones, B. (1991). Dysphagia occurring after polio. *Dysphagia, 6,* 165–169.

Bushman, M., Dobmeyer, S.M., Leeker, L., & Perlmutter, J.S. (1989). Swallowing abnormalities and their response to treatment in Parkinson's disease. *Neurology, 39,* 1309–1314.

Butcher, R.B. (1982). Treatment of chronic aspiration as complication of cerebrovascular accident. *Laryngoscope, 92,* 681–685.

Calne, D.B., Shaw, D.G., Spiers, A.S.D., & Stern, G.M. (1970). Swallowing in Parkinsonism. *British Journal of Radiology, 43,* 456–457.

Carpenter, R.J., McDonald, T.J., & Howard, F.M. (1978). The otolaryngologic presentation of amyotrophic lateral sclerosis. *Otolaryngology, 86,* 479–484.

Casey, E., & Aminoff, M. (1971). Dystrophia myotonica presenting with dysphagia. *British Medical Journal, 2,* 443.

Celifarco, A., Gerard, G., Faegenburg, D., & Burakoff, R. (1990). Dysphagia as the sole manifestation of bilateral strokes. *The American Journal of Gastroenterology, 85,* 610–613.

Chen, M.Y.M., Ott, D.J., Peele, V.N., & Gelfand, D. (1990). Oropharynx in patients with cerebrovascular disease: Evaluation with videofluroscopy. *Radiology, 176,* 641–643.

Cherney, L.R. (in press). Speech and swallowing disorders. In J.E. Morley (Ed.), *Geriatric medicine.* St. Louis: The Manning Company.

Cherney, L.R., & Halper, A.S. (1989). Recovery of oral nutrition after head injury in adults. *Journal of Head Trauma Rehabilitation, 4* (4), 42–50.

Coelho, C.A., & Ferranti, R. (1988). Dysphagia in postpolio sequelae: Report of three cases. *Archives of Physical Medicine and Rehabilitation, 69,* 634–636.

Coelho, C.A., & Ferranti, R. (1991). Incidence and nature of dysphagia in polio survivors. *Archives of Physical Medicine and Rehabilitation, 72,* 1071–1075.

Cummings, J.L., & Benson, D.F. (1983). *Dementia: A clinical approach.* Boston: Butterworth.

Daly, D.C., Code, C.F., & Anderson, H.A. (1962). Disturbances of swallowing and esophageal motility in patients with multiple sclerosis. *Neurology, 12,* 250–256.

Darley, F.L., Aronson, A.E., & Brown, J.R. (1975). *Motor Speech Disorders,* Philadelphia: W.B. Saunders.

Dodds, W.J. (1989). The physiology of swallowing, *Dysphagia, 3,* 171–178.

Dodds, W.J., Logemann, J.A., & Stewart, E.T. (1990a). Physiology and radiology of normal oral and pharyngeal phases of swallowing. *American Journal of Radiology, 154,* 953–963.

Dodds, W.J., Stewart, E.T., & Logemann, J.A. (1990b). Radiologic assessment of abnormal oral and pharyngeal phases of swallowing. *American Journal of Radiology, 154,* 965–974.

Donner, M. (1974). Swallowing mechanism and neuromuscular disorder. *Seminars in Roentgenology, 9,* 273–282.

Doty, R.W. (1968). Neural organization of deglutition. In C.F. Code (Ed.), *Handbook of physiology, IV* (pp. 1861–1902). Washington, DC: American Physiological Society.

Duranceau, C., Leterdre, J., Clemont, R., Levesque, H., & Barbeau, A. (1978). Oropharyngeal dysphagia in patients with oculopharyngeal muscular dystrophy. *Canadian Journal of Surgery, 21,* 326–329.

Dworkin, J.P., & Hartman, D.E. (1979). Progressive deterioration and dysphagia in amyotrophic lateral sclerosis: Case report. *Archives of Physical Medicine and Rehabilitation, 60,* 423–425.

Eadie, M.J., & Tyrer, J.H. (1965). Alimentary disorders in Parkinsonism. *Australian Annals of Medicine, 14,* 13–22.

Ekberg, O., & Feinberg, M.J. (1991). Altered swallowing function in elderly patients without dysphagia: Radiologic findings in 56 cases. *American Journal of Radiology, 156,* 1181–1184.

Feinberg, M. J., & Ekberg, O. (1991). Videofluorographic evaluation of oropharyngeal function in dementia. *Dysphagia, 6,* 181.

Field, L.H., & Weiss, C.J. (1989). Dysphagia with head injury. *Brain Injury, 3,* 19–26.

Fischer, R.A., Ellison, G.W., Thayer, W.R., Spiro, H.M., & Glaser, G.H. (1965). Esophageal motility in neuromuscular disorders. *Annals of Internal Medicine, 63,* 229–248.

Gordon, C., Hewer, R.L., & Wade, D.T. (1987). Dysphagia in acute stroke. *British Medical Journal, 295,* 411–414.

Greenspan, D., & Greenspan, J.S. (1988). The oral features of HIV infection. *Gastroenterology Clinics of North America, 17,* 535–543.

Gresham, S.L. (1990). Clinical assessment and management of swallowing difficulties after stroke. *The Medical Journal of Australia, 153,* 397–399.

Groher, M.E., (1991). *The clinical and research implications of AIDS for the speech/language pathologist.* Paper presented at the American Speech Language Hearing Association Annual Convention, Meeting of the Special Interest Division: Neurophysiology and Neurogenic Speech and Language Disorders, Atlanta, GA.

Groher, M.E., & Bukatman, R. (1986). The prevalence of swallowing in two teaching hospitals. *Dysphagia, 1,* 3–6.

Groher, M.E., & Gonzalez, E.E. (1992). Mechanical disorders of swallowing. In M.E. Groher (Ed.), *Dysphagia: Diagnosis and management* (2nd ed.). Boston: Butterworth-Heinemann.

Hellemans, J., Pelemans, W., & Van Trappen, G. (1981). Pharyngoesophageal swallowing disorders and the pharyngoesophageal sphincter. *Medical Clinics of North America, 65,* (6), 1149–1171.

Herrera, W., Zeligman, B.E., Gruber, J., Jones, M.C., Pautler, R., Wriston, R., Cain, M., Prescott, T., Cobble, N., & Burks, J.S. (1990). Dysphagia in multiple sclerosis: Clinical and videofluoroscopic correlations. *Journal of Neurologic Rehabilitation, 4,* 1–8.

Hillel, A.D., & Miller, R.M. (1989). Bulbar amyotrophic lateral sclerosis: Patterns of progression and clinical management. *Head and Neck, 11,* 51–59.

Horner, J., Buoyer, F.G., Alberts, M.J., & Helms, M.J. (1991). Dysphagia following brain-stem stroke: Clinical correlates and outcome. *Archives of Neurology, 48,* 1170–1173.

Horner, J., Massey, E.W., & Brazer, S.R. (1990). Dysphagia after bilateral stroke. *Neurology, 40,* 1686–1688.

Hughes, C.V., Baum, B.J., Fox, P.C., Marmary, Y., Yeh, C.K., & Sonies, B.C. (1987). Oral-pharyngeal dysphagia: A common sequela of salivary gland dysfunction. *Dysphagia, 1,* 173–177.

Johnson, E.R., McKenzie, S.W., Rosenquist, C.J., Lieberman, J.S., & Sievers, A.E. (1992). Dysphagia following stroke: Quantitative evaluation of pharyngeal transit times. *Archives of Physical Medicine and Rehabilitation, 73,* 419–423.

Jones, B., Bucholz, D.W., Ravich, W.J., & Donner, M.W. (1992). Swallowing dysfunction in the postpolio syndrome: A cinefluorographic study. *American Journal of Radiology, 158,* 283–286.

Kagel, M.C., & Leopold, N.A. (1992). Dysphagia in Huntington's disease: A 16-year retrospective. *Dysphagia, 7,* 106–114.

Kahrilas, P.J., Dodds, W., Dent, J., Logemann, J., & Shaker, R. (1988). Upper esophageal sphincter function during deglutition. *Gastroenterology, 95,* 52–62.

Klawans, H.K., & Tanner, C.M. (1984). Movement disorders in the elderly. In M.L. Albert (Ed.), *Clinical neurology of aging.* New York: Oxford University Press.

Langmore, S.E. (1991). Managing the complications of aspiration in dysphagic adults. *Seminars in Speech and Language, 12* (3), 199–208.

Layne, K.A., Losinski, D.S., Zenner, P.M., & Ament, J.A. (1989). Using the Fleming index of dysphagia to establish prevalence. *Dysphagia, 4,* 39–42.

Lazarus, C., & Logemann, J.A. (1987). Swallowing disorders in closed head trauma patients. *Archives of Physical Medicine and Rehabilitation, 68,* 79–84.

Lazzara, G., Lazarus, C., & Logemann, J.A. (1985). Swallowing disorders in spinal cord injured patients. *ASHA, 27,* 123.

Leopold, N.A., & Kagel, M.C. (1975). Dysphagia in Huntington's disease. *Archives of Neurology, 42,* 57–60.

Leopold, N.A., & Kagel, M.C. (1983). Swallowing ingestion and dysphagia: A reappraisal. *Archives of Physical Medicine and Rehabilitation, 64,* 371–373.

Lieberman, A.M., Horowitz, L., Redmond, P., Pachter, L., Lieberman, I., & Leibowitz, M. (1980). Dysphagia in Parkinson's disease. *American Journal of Gastroenterology, 74,* 157–160.

Logemann, J.A. (1983). *Evaluation and treatment of swallowing disorders.* San Diego: College Hill Press.

Logemann, J.A. (1985). The relationship of speech and swallowing in head and neck surgical patients. *Seminars in Speech and Language, 6,* 351–359.

Logemann, J.A. (1986). Treatment for aspiration related to dysphagia: An overview. *Dysphagia, 1,* 34–38.

Logemann, J.A. (1988). Swallowing physiology and pathophysiology. *Otolaryngologic Clinics of North America, 21,* 613–623.

Logemann, J.A. (1990). Factors affecting ability to resume oral nutrition in the oropharyngeal dysphagic individual. *Dysphagia, 4,* 202–208.

Logemann, J.A., Blonsky, E., & Boshes, B. (1975). Dysphagia in Parkinsonism. *Journal of the American Medical Association, 231,* 69–70.

Logemann, J.A., Kahrilas, P.J., Cheng, J., Pauloski, B.R., Gibbons, P.J., Rademaker, A.W., & Lin, S. (1992). Closure mechanisms of laryngeal vestibule during swallow. *American Journal of Physiology, 262,* G337–G344.

Ludman, H. (1962). Dysphagia in dystrophia myotonica. *Journal of Laryngology, 76,* 234–236.

Martin, B.J.W. 1994. Treatment of dysphagia in adults. In L.R. Cherney (Ed.), *Clinical management of dysphagia.* Gaithersburg, MD: Aspen Publishers, Inc.

McConnell, F.M.S., Cerenko, D., Jackson, R.T., & Guffin, T.N. (1988). Timing of major events of pharyngeal swallowing. *Archives of Otolaryngology and Head and Neck Surgery, 114,* 1413–1418.

Meadows, J. (1973). Dysphagia in unilateral cerebral lesions. *Journal of Neurology, Neurosurgery, and Psychiatry, 36,* 853–860.

Miller, A.J. (1982). Deglutition. *Physiological Review, 62,* 129–184.

Miller, A.J. (1986). Neurophysiological basis of swallowing. *Dysphagia, 1,* 91–100.

Miller, R.M., & Groher, M.E. (1982). The evaluation and management of neuromuscular and mechanical swallowing disorders. *Dysarthria, Dysphonia, Dysphagia, 1,* 50–70.

Miller, R.M., & Groher, M.E. (1992). General treatment of neurologic swallowing disorders. In M.E. Groher (Ed.), *Dysphagia: Diagnosis and management,* 2nd ed., pp. 197–217. Stoneham, MA: Butterworth-Heinemann.

Morrell, R.M. (1992). Neurologic disorders of swallowing. In M.E. Groher (Ed.), *Dysphagia: Diagnosis and management,* 2nd ed., pp. 31–51. Stoneham, MA: Butterworth–Heinemann.

Murray, J.P. (1962). Deglutition in myasthenia gravis. *British Journal of Radiology, 35,* 43–52.

Nowack, W., Hatelid, J., & Sohn, R. (1977). Dysphagia in Parkinsonism. *Archives of Neurology, 34,* 320.

Palmer, E.D. (1974). Dysphagia in Parkinsonism. *Journal of the American Medical Association, 29,* 1349.

Pannell, J.J., Cantieri, C.A., & Cherney, L.R. (1984). *Evaluation of dysphagia in the neurologically impaired.* Poster presented at the meeting of the Illinois Speech Language and Hearing Association, Chicago.

Perlman, A.L. (1991). The neurology of swallowing. *Seminars in Speech and Language, 12,* 171–184.

Pierce, J.W., Creamer, B., & MacDermot, V. (1965). Abnormalities in swallowing associated with dystrophia myotonica. *Gut, 6,* 392–395.

Rabeneck, L., Popovic, M., Gartner, S., McLean, D.M., McLeod, W.A., Read, E., Wong, K.K., & Boyko, W.J. (1990). Acute HIV infection presenting with painful swallowing and esophageal ulcers. *Journal of the American Medical Association, 263* (17), 2318.

Raufman, J.P. (1988). Odynophagia/dysphagia in AIDS. *Gastroenterology Clinics of North America, 17,* 599–614.

Robbins, J. (1987). Swallowing in ALS and motor neuron disorders. *Neurologic Clinics, 5,* 213–229.

Robbins, J., Hamilton, J.W., Lof, G.L., & Kempster, G.B. (1992). Oropharyngeal swallowing in normal adults of different ages. *Gastroenterology, 103,* 823–829.

Robbins, J., & Levine, R. (1988). Swallowing after unilateral stroke of the cerebral cortex. *Dysphagia, 3,* 11–17.

Robbins, J., Logemann, J.A., & Kirshner, H.S. (1986). Swallowing and speech production in Parkinson's disease. *Annals of Neurology, 19,* 283–287.

Sheth, N., & Diner, W.C. (1988). Swallowing problems in the elderly. *Dysphagia, 2,* 209–215.

Siebens, H., Trupe, E., Siebens, A., Cook, F., Anshen, S., Hanauer, R., & Oster, G. (1986). Correlates and consequences of eating dependency in institutionalized elderly. *Journal of the American Geriatric Society, 34,* 192–198.

Silbergleit, A.K., Waring, W.P., Sullivan, M.J., & Maynard, F.M. (1991). Evaluation, treatment, and follow-up results of post-polio patients with dysphagia. *Otolaryngology Head and Neck Surgery, 104,* 333–338.

Silbiger, M.L., Pikielney, R., & Donner, M.W. (1967). Neuromuscular disorders affecting the pharynx: Cineradiographic analysis. *Investigative Radiology, 2,* 442–448.

Singer, E.J. (1991). Central nervous system (CNS) sequelae of HIV disease. American Speech Language Hearing Association, Special Interest Division 2. *Neurophysiology and Neurogenic Speech and Language Disorders, 1* (2), 2–7.

Sonies, B.C. (1987). Oral-motor problems. In Mueller, H.G., & Geoffrey, V.C. (Eds.), *Communication disorders and aging: Assessment and management,* pp. 185–213. Washington, DC: Gallaudet University Press.

Sonies, B.C. (1992a). Oropharyngeal dysphagia in the elderly. *Clinics in Geriatric Medicine, 8,* 569–577.

Sonies, B.C. (1992b). Speech and swallowing in progressive supranuclear palsy. In I. Litvan & Y. Agid (Eds.), *Progressive supranuclear palsy: Clinical and research approaches.* pp. 240–253. New York: Oxford University Press.

Sonies, B.C., & Dalakas, M.C. (1991). Dysphagia in patients with the post-polio syndrome. *The New England Journal of Medicine, 324,* 1162–1167.

Sonies, B.C., Parent, L.J., Morrish, K., & Baum, B.J. (1988). Durational aspects of the oral-pharyngeal phase of swallow in normal adults. *Dysphagia, 3,* 1–10.

Stroudley, J., & Walsh, M. (1991). Radiologic assessment of dysphagia in Parkinson's disease. *British Journal of Radiology, 64,* 890–893.

Tippett, D.C., Palmer, J., & Linden, P. (1987). Management of dysphagia in a patient with closed head injury. *Dysphagia, 1,* 221–226.

Tracy, J.F., Logemann, J.A., & Kahrilas, P.J. (1989a). Dysphagia following cervical spine injury: Patterns of recovery. *ASHA, 31,* 108.

Tracy, J.F., Logemann, J.A., Kahrilas, P.J., Jacob, P., Kobara, M., & Krugler, C. (1989b). Preliminary observations on the effects of age on oropharyngeal deglutition. *Dysphagia, 4,* 90–94.

Veis, S., & Logemann, J. (1985). Swallowing disorders in persons with cerebrovascular accident. *Archives of Physical Medicine and Rehabilitation, 66,* 372–375.

Veis, S., & Logemann, J.A. (1991). Dysphagia after spinal cord injury. *ASHA, 33,* 112.

Winstein, C.J. (1983). Frequency, progression, and outcome in adults following head injury. *Physical Therapy, 63,* 1992–1997.

Wyse, M., Grant, M., & Redenbaugh, M. (1984). Dysphagia management following right cerebral vascular accident: Behavioral considerations. *ASHA, 26,* 83.

Young, E.C., & Durant-Jones, L. (1990). Developing a dysphagia program in an acute care hospital: A needs assessment. *Dysphagia, 5,* 159–165.

◆ CHAPTER 2 ◆

Oral-Motor and Swallowing Skills in the Infant and Child: An Overview

Maureen M. Boner and Wendy S. Perlin

NORMAL DEVELOPMENT OF ORAL-MOTOR/SWALLOWING SKILLS

It is often too easy to think of the eating process in terms of the oral mechanism only. Eating is a complex process that includes levels of alertness, cognition, motor and neurologic development, bonding to the caregiver, and physiologic maturation of the system. Many of these skills begin *in utero* and develop through early childhood.

Prenatal Period

Various sources state that fetal swallowing begins as early as 11 weeks gestation (Weiss, 1988), whereas others indicate that it begins at 16 to 17 weeks gestation (Grand, Watkins, & Torti, 1976; Pritchard, 1966; Tuchman, 1989). All agree that fetal swallowing aids in the management of amniotic fluid volume. By term (40 weeks), the fetus is swallowing 450 mL/day, or nearly one-half of the total volume of amniotic fluid (Committee on Nutrition, American Academy of Pediatrics, 1985; Tuchman, 1988). Sucking develops at 27 to 28 weeks gestation but is not mature until approximately 30 to 34 weeks. Therefore, most practitioners advise that working on sucking with premature infants whose gestational age is less than 30 to 34 weeks is inappropriate. These infants are not neurologically equipped for sucking (Committee on Nutrition, American Academy of Pediatrics, 1985).

Postnatal Period

Feeding development consists of maturation and integration of all components necessary for normal eating. The postnatal developmental process is separated into three periods by the American College of Pediatrics: the *nursing period*, the *transitional period,* and the *modified adult period* (Committee on Nutrition, American Academy of Pediatrics, 1985).

Nursing Period

Nutrition

During the nursing period, from birth to 4 to 6 months of age, the infant takes in human milk or milk-based formula. One to two percent of all children demonstrate an intolerance to milk-based formulas. The current hypothesis is that these intolerances are a manifestation of either a protein hypersensitivity or a lactose intolerance (Committee on Nutrition, American Academy of Pediatrics, 1985). Whole cow's milk should not be given to any infant until at least 6 months of age (Committee on Nutrition, American Academy of Pediatrics, 1985). It contains little iron, linoleic acid, and vitamin C. Children fed primarily with cow's milk at an early age often present with iron deficiency, anemia, and bleeding from the gastrointestinal tract (Committee on Nutrition, American Academy of Pediatrics, 1985).

Premature infants present with different nutritional needs. Their nitrogen and mineral requirements are higher per unit weight than those of a full-term infant. However, nature appears to compensate for this, as studies show that the breast milk from mothers of premature infants has 10 to 30 percent more nitrogen, sodium, chlorine, and magnesium than the milk of a mother after the delivery of a full-term infant (Committee on Nutrition, American Academy of Pediatrics, 1985).

During the nursing period, the infant can suck(le) only liquids. The intestinal tract has not developed a defense mechanism to cope with foreign proteins. The kidneys are not mature enough to handle the large osmolar loads of proteins and electrolytes. It is common for infants to lose weight after birth. However, the original birth weight should be regained by 3 weeks of age. No additional weight should be lost after 10 days of age (Committee on Nutrition, American Academy of Pediatrics, 1985).

Development

  Birth to 3 Months:

  1. *Primitive Reflexes:* Normal infants are born with a set of reflexes that are basic to survival. Most of these reflexes are assimilated as the infant develops more control over his or her body and the environment. Children who are neurologically impaired may continue to exhibit these reflexes beyond the normal developmental stage. The persistence of these reflexes interferes with the child's development in all areas, including feeding and swallowing. Exhibit 2-1 describes and summarizes these primitive reflexes.

Exhibit 2-1 Primitive Reflexes

- **Rooting** is a primitive reflex that aids the infant in finding the source of nutrition. When the corner of the infant's mouth is touched, the infant turns toward the source searching for the nipple or bottle. Rooting is present from birth to 3 months but is retained longer by breast-fed infants (Alexander, 1988).

- The **transverse tongue** reflex is stimulated by touch or taste on the lateral portion of the tongue. This reflex causes the tongue to move in the direction of the stimulus. It is evident from birth to 6 months of age.

- The **bite** reflex is also present from birth to 6 months. This is a rhythmic series of up-and-down jaw movements produced after tactile stimulation to the teeth or gums.

- The **gag** reflex is present from birth throughout life. However, some sources cite as many as 40 percent of normal adults do not exhibit a gag reflex (Logemann, 1990). Stimulation to the posterior half of the oral cavity results in mouth opening, head extension, and the floor of the mouth depressing (Bailey & Wolery, 1989).

- The **asymmetric tonic neck reflex (ATNR)**, also known as the "fencer's position," is present from birth to 4 months of age. To stimulate this reflex, place the child in supine. Turn the child's head to the side and watch for extension of the arm on the child's face side and flexion of the arm on the skull side. This is normally present bilaterally.

- The **Babkin** occurs when deep pressure is applied to the palm of the infant's hand. This results in the infant opening his or her mouth, closing the eyes, and bringing the head forward.

- The **palmomental** reflex is elicited by touching the palm of the hand, causing the chin to wrinkle.

- The **grasp** is elicited as the adult places his or her finger across the palm of the infant, giving a slight pull. The baby responds by grasping and holding onto the finger.

- The **startle** reflex is present at birth and is elicited by pushing the child backward in supported sitting or by making a loud noise. The child reflexively extends and abducts arms and legs.

Babkin, grasp, palmomental, and **startle** reflexes are of little importance to survival or development of oral/motor skills (Morris & Klein, 1987). However, they do influence the future development of self-feeding skills. Each of these is present from birth to 3 months of age.

2. *Feeding:* In the period from birth to 3 months, the infant's lips approximate the nipple but are not actively closed. Some loss of liquid may be noted. There is active suckling with some intermittent sucking. The tongue is held in a cupped configuration with central grooving to move food back for the swallow. The swallow is accomplished with a small amount of tongue protrusion. There is wide jaw excursion, and some asymmetry may be noted. The rooting reflex is present until about 3 months. The baby's intake is infant formula or breast milk, taken in short bursts of two to three sucks before pausing. Although there is variance between children, 2 to 6 ounces are taken per feeding every 2 to 4 hours.

3. *Respiration:* Infants are nasal breathers until approximately 3 months of age, because the epiglottis actually comes in contact with the soft palate (Weiss, 1988). Breathing is asynchronous and fluctuates between belly-breathing and upper-chest breathing. During respiration, the thoracic cavity depresses, the abdomen expands, and occasional sternal notching may be seen. This occurs because of the strong pull of the diaphragm without any other active muscle control to counterbalance the action (McGee, 1987).

4. *Speech and Language:* In newborns, vocal productions usually consist of open vowels produced during crying episodes. Vegetative sounds are produced during eating (Alexander, 1988). Toward the end of this period, a differentiated cry develops. Some cooing may be evident, but it is typically heard with associated body movement. With further development, pitch and intonation start to vary (Alexander, 1988).

Four to Six Months:

1. *Feeding:* Lips begin to show active movement, as the upper lip closes over a spoon. The lower lip is often indrawn when the spoon is removed. Suckling disappears and is replaced by an active suck. The child is able to take 20 or more successive sucks. The suck-swallow is coordinated so that the child rarely needs to pause for a breath. No liquid is lost from the bottle or breast. The tongue base is more stabilized, with excursion remaining within the mouth. Tongue movement accompanies jaw movement. Jaw excursion is reduced. There is visual recognition of the spoon or bottle. Primary nutrition is still achieved by breast milk or formula. The baby is able to take 8 to 10 oz per feeding, usually every 4 to 6 hours. Most pediatricians recommend solid foods (pureed foods) be introduced at 6 months of age or older. However, rice cereals are often introduced at an earlier age through bottle or spoon.

2. *Respiration:* In the 6-month-old infant, more thoracic breathing is noted. He or she spends more time in an upright position and is developing abdominal muscle control (McGee, 1987).

3. *Speech and Language:* By 6 months of age, facial expressions begin to vary and laughter is heard. The infant's cry becomes significantly differentiated with increased jaw stabilization. More sustained and less nasalized vowels are produced. Some consonant/vowel combinations are produced with the eruption of the infant's first teeth. The infant also starts to imitate some sounds, and babbling begins to emerge (McGee, 1987).

Swallowing

The method by which the infant manipulates the bolus and swallows is highly contrasted against the adult swallow (Bosma, 1978). Few studies have been completed on infant swallowing because of ethical issues surrounding the exposure of normal children during radiographic studies. However, theories are being formed based on differences in physiology, neurologic maturation, clinical observations, and information gained from videofluoroscopic studies in children with actual or suspected swallowing problems (Logemann, 1990).

Anatomically, the oral and pharyngeal cavities in an infant are both "absolutely and proportionately smaller" (Logemann, 1990). The oral cavity is smaller but also filled completely by the tongue. Early in development, the entire tongue is in the oral cavity. Later, it drops so that the base becomes part of the pharyngeal wall. Buccal cheek pads or "fatpads" fill the lateral sulci and further reduce the size of the oral cavity. Because of this, nasal breathing is essential. In the pharyngeal and laryngeal cavities, the larynx and hyoid bone are elevated with little space between them (Bosma, 1978). The epiglottis is larger and omega-shaped. The pyriform sinuses are smaller and elevated, and the arytenoid cartilages are larger. The wall of the soft palate and the tongue base are closer together. Figure 2-1 compares the anatomy of the infant and adult. Because of the relative positions of structures in infants and the relatively small amount of active movement/control in the process, the infant is set to take nutrition in an efficient manner with relatively little expenditure of energy. Therefore, mild neurologic deficits may remain undetected until further maturation, when structural protection is no longer present (Logemann, 1990).

The normal process of swallowing begins with first contact of the nipple to the lips. Infants use repeated tongue and/or jaw pumping to express liquid from the nipple. Little or no active sucking is required. With compression of the jaw, the anterior portion of the tongue elevates, squeezing the milk from the nipple while the back of the tongue is depressed, leaving a space for the milk to collect (Bu'Lock, Woolridge, & Baum, 1990). Tongue elevation moves in a wave-like motion until the anterior portion is depressed and the posterior portion of the tongue is elevated, pressing against the soft palate and theoretically holding the bolus before initiation of the pharyngeal swallow (Bu'Lock et al., 1990). During this process, the small oral cavity, filled by the tongue and fatpads, is expanded through jaw opening, causing a vacuum to develop, which further aids posterior movement of the liquid (Bu'lock et al., 1990). There is current debate regarding location of bolus collection before initiation of the swallow. In adults, the bolus is collected anterior to the soft palate at the faucial arches. Logemann (1990) has described collection in the valleculae before initiation of the swallow in children who present with no other "abnormalities." She suggested that this may be an acceptable developmental pattern that matures to adult level by the time adult chewing is stabilized (approximately 2 1/2 to 3 years of age).

Regardless of site of bolus collection, the tongue base and pharyngeal wall come together, creating negative pressure below and driving the bolus down. There is forward movement of the larynx, causing the esophageal sphincter to open. Laryngeal elevation is minimal, as the larynx and hyoid

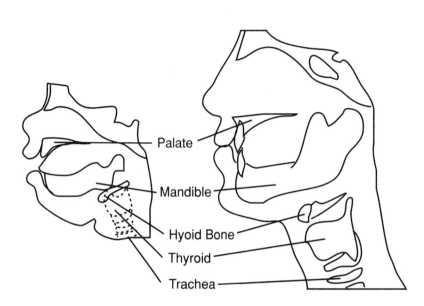

Figure 2-1 Infant Anatomy. *Source:* From "Special swallowing problems in children" by S. Kramer, 1985, *Gastrointestinal Radiology, 10*, p. 243. Copyright 1985 by Springer-Verlag. Reprinted by permission.

are already elevated and close to one another. With forward laryngeal movement, the epiglottis moves forward, widening the path to the esophagus. Simultaneously, cricopharyngeal opening occurs. As the relatively large arytenoid cartilages tilt forward, they close the vocal folds and theoretically add more airway protection (Logemann, 1990). During a fraction of a second, breathing is stopped (Tuchman, 1988). The bolus travels into the esophagus and is carried to the stomach through peristaltic movement.

As soon as the suck-hold breath-swallow cycle is completed, it is reactivated. Coordination between these components is essential.

Transitional Period

Nutrition

In the transitional period, from 4 to 6 months to 1 year of age, the infant ingests specially prepared food in addition to human milk and formula. Neuromuscular mechanisms needed for recognizing a spoon, masticating, and swallowing nonliquid foods are developing. Therefore, the infant is able to indicate a desire for food by opening his or her mouth and leaning forward. Disinterest is indicated by turning away. The infant enjoys variation in taste and color of the food. The intestines have developed more mature defense mechanisms and can digest and absorb more proteins, fats, and carbohydrates. The kidneys can now handle osmolar loads with less water. The introduction of solid foods should begin with single-ingredient foods, presented one at a time at weekly intervals. This will allow the caregiver to determine food intolerance. A combination of foods, cereal, and fruit may be given after tolerance for individual components is established. The healthy infant rarely requires additional water except in hot weather. However, after the introduction of solid foods, increased water is needed because the renal osmolar load is high in foods with higher protein or electrolyte content (i.e., meats, egg yolk). It is during this period that whole cow's milk is generally introduced (Committee on Nutrition, American Academy of Pediatrics, 1985).

Development

Seven to Nine Months:

1. *Feeding:* Lips are more active in the sucking process. Actual pull on the nipple is noted. Solid foods (pureed and, later, soft chopped) are introduced. The upper lip may assist in removal of food from the spoon. The tongue is able to move thicker and drier food posteriorly for swallowing. The child is able to collect several pieces of food into one bolus and can place and replace food onto gums or teeth for breaking apart. Sensory feedback is given to the temporo-mandibular joint (TMJ) and the gums in the act of eating. Facial muscles give feedback to the jaw regarding pressure readings that contribute to increased jaw control and grading. Tongue protrusion may be evident. Chewing reflexes begin, and the child begins to bite off crackers, using a phasic bite. Some lateral tongue movement is seen. No loss of liquid is noted in bottle or breast feeding after 6 months of age. Cup drinking is accomplished with a mixture of sucking and suckling patterns. Wide jaw excursions and loss of liquid are often seen. Drooling is controlled, except when teething, mouthing hands and toys, or when babbling. During this period, infants generally take 11 oz or more of fluid per feeding (Committee on Nutrition, American Academy of Pediatrics, 1985).

2. *Respiration:* Greater thoracic breathing is noted as the child begins to use upper and lower trunk rotation (McGee, 1987).

3. *Speech and Language:* The infant displays an increase in reduplicated syllables, tongue clicks, and "raspberries" in play. Chains of consonants are produced frequently. The infant vocalizes similar sound patterns after hearing them. First spontaneous words may emerge (Alexander, 1988).

Nine to Twelve Months:

1. *Feeding:* Both lips are active in food removal from the spoon. The child now demonstrates good pressure control of the tongue. The tongue tip begins to elevate, dissociating from the jaw. There is emerging lateral and diagonal jaw and tongue movement. The child is able to hold and bite a soft cookie or cracker. He or she may have more difficulty with harder foods. The lips and cheeks continue learning pressure control. The child may begin cleaning the lips with the tongue. He or she drinks from a cup, taking 2 to 3 sips before pausing for a breath. Some jaw stability is achieved by biting on the cup edge or by slight tongue protrusion under the rim of the cup. Some liquid may be lost. No drooling is seen during gross motor activities and movements.

2. *Respiration:* More thoracic movement is noted with inhalation. Breathing is more synchronous than it was in earlier stages (Alexander, 1988).
3. *Speech and Language:* Jargon and first words develop. The infant plays at making different sounds and sound patterns. Variation in intonation and pitch is evident. The infant imitates new words, although the imitations are not always accurate (Alexander, 1988).

Swallowing

During this developmental period, it becomes easier to discriminate the swallowing phases (preparatory, oral, pharyngeal, and esophageal). The normal swallowing process appears to mature to a near-adult level between the ages of 2 and 3 years (Morris & Klein, 1987). This process is described in Chapter 1.

Modified Adult Period

Nutrition

In the modified adult period, from 12 to 24 months of age, most nutrients come from regular table foods. Physiologic mechanisms have matured to near-adult levels of proficiency. The infant is learning to self-feed. Table food is cut into small pieces. The infant is developing specific taste discrimination and preferences.

Development

Twelve to Eighteen Months:

1. *Feeding:* Lip, tongue, and jaw movements are independent of one another. Tongue tip refinement is noted, and diagonal tongue movement is seen. There is tongue tip stabilization during the swallow. The child cleans his or her lips by scraping them across teeth or gums. A controlled bite is present. Lateral and vertical jaw movements combine to form a beginning rotary chew. The child is able to chew with his or her mouth open. Toward the end of this period, the child chews meat with some difficulty.
2. *Respiration:* Respiratory patterns do not change during this period.
3. *Speech and Language:* The child produces single words (10 to 15) spontaneously. He or she imitates new words and increases the consonant repertoire to include *d*, *t*, *n*, and *h* (Rossetti, 1990).

Eighteen to Twenty-Four Months:

1. *Feeding:* No drooling is seen, even during fine motor tasks. All textures are eaten. Tongue tip pointing and thinning are seen. Rotary chew continues to develop.
2. *Respiration:* Respiratory patterns do not change during this period.
3. *Speech and Language:* The child uses 50 words spontaneously. Two-word phrases are produced and new words are used regularly (Rossetti, 1990).

Swallowing

By this time, the process of swallowing is established and remains the same throughout adulthood. Some refinement in control may be seen.

FEEDING AND SWALLOWING DYSFUNCTION ASSOCIATED WITH SPECIFIC DISORDERS

There are many congenital and acquired disorders that result in feeding and swallowing problems. Feeding and swallowing problems may result directly from an injury or may occur as an associated problem, secondary to the injury. The following compilation summarizes the most frequently occurring characteristics cited in the literature and seen clinically. The extent to which characteristics are displayed depends on where the normal developmental process was interrupted (be it congenital or acquired later in life), site and severity of the lesion, and the amount of spontaneous recovery. *Each child will present with a different profile and will not necessarily display all the characteristics listed below.* Some children who do not present with a neurologic basis for feeding problems display immature feeding patterns. These patterns may result from prolonged nonoral feeding, lack of oral motor stimulation, and/or behavioral problems (Ylvisaker & Weinstein, 1989).

Cerebral Palsy

A variety of feeding and swallowing problems may accompany cerebral palsy depending on the type of muscle tone, presence of primitive reflexes, movement patterns, and the integrity of the sensory system (Bailey & Wolery, 1989; McGee, 1987). Current studies on children with cerebral palsy are limited in number of subjects and do not always differentiate the different types of cerebral palsy. In general, studies cite poor lingual control and delay in the pharyngeal swallow, which may result in aspiration (Griggs, Jones, & Lee, 1989; Helfrich-Miller, Rector, & Straka, 1986; Logemann, 1983) and reduced pharyngeal peristalsis (Logemann, 1983).

The sensory motor problems interfere with sensation and physical control during the eating process. Cognitive and language problems may also complicate the eating process (Jones, 1989). The feeding process is often inefficient and lengthy. Therefore, many of these children present with poor nutritional intake (Griggs et al., 1989).

The most frequently-occurring types of cerebral palsy are listed below.

1. *Spastic Cerebral Palsy*

General Characteristics	*Related Feeding Characteristics*
• Increased tone • Decreased range of motion	• Loss of food/liquid secondary to poor lip closure and poor lingual control (Griggs, et al., 1989)

1. *Spastic Cerebral Palsy* (continued)

General Characteristics

- Shallow respiration/decreased ribcage mobility (McGee, 1987)
- Compensatory posturing
- Cognitive deficits (Levitt, 1982)
- Perceptual problems (Levitt, 1982)
- Seizure disorder (Levitt, 1982)

Related Feeding Characteristics

- Flattened, retracted tongue
- Retracted lips
- Decreased bolus formation
- Decreased control of bolus secondary to poor lingual mobility (Griggs et al., 1989)
- Increased oral transit time
- Difficulty managing very thick or very thin textures
- Inadequate velopharyngeal closure
- Possible structural abnormalities (high-arched palate)
- Inability to breathe through nose while sucking
- Poor jaw control
- Delay in pharyngeal swallow (Logemann, 1983)
- Reduced pharyngeal peristalsis (Griggs et al., 1989)
- Compensatory posturing during feeding
- Drooling
- Lower respiratory infections secondary to aspiration (Griggs et al., 1989; Jones, 1989)

2. *Athetoid Cerebral Palsy*

General Characteristics

- Fluctuating tone
- Inconsistent breathing patterns
- Poor head control
- Difficulty maintaining optimal positioning (McGee, 1987)

Related Feeding Characteristics

- Loss of food or liquid secondary to poor lip closure
- Retraction of lower lip (McGee, 1987)
- Facial grimace

2. *Athetoid Cerebral Palsy* (continued)

General Characteristics

- Involuntary movement patterns (Levitt, 1982)
- Writhing/athetoid movements
- Difficulty isolating eye movements from head movement (Connor, Williamson, & Siepp, 1978)
- Possible cognitive deficits

Related Feeding Characteristics

- Poor coordination of lip and tongue movement
- Inability to coordinate breathing and sucking
- Poor manipulation of bolus
- Drooling

3. *Ataxic Cerebral Palsy*

General Characteristics

- Generally decreased tone (Connor et al., 1978)
- Imprecise direction of movement
- Over- and undershooting movements
- May have athetoid and/or spastic components (McGee, 1987)
- Poor balance and coordination (Connor et al., 1978)
- Postural fixation
- Nystagmus (Levitt, 1982)
- Possible cognitive deficits (Levitt, 1982)
- Perceptual deficits (Levitt, 1982)

Related Feeding Characteristics

- Loss of food/liquid secondary to poor lip closure
- Inconsistent poor coordination of breathing and eating/drinking
- May present with any combination of feeding patterns listed under spastic or athetoid cerebral palsy (McGee, 1987)
- Drooling

Traumatic Brain Injury

The following characteristics are typical of children who have sustained a traumatic brain injury. Characteristics vary widely depending on the stage of recovery and the site(s) of injury. Some direct effect on feeding skills may be seen, such as dysarthria and swallowing problems.

However, many of the problems are secondary to decreased cognition, orientation, alertness, attention, and abnormal muscle tone.

<table>
<tr><td>

General Characteristics

- Increased agitation
- Abnormal sensation: hyper- and hyposensitivity (Ylvisaker & Logemann, 1985)
- Poor initiation (Logemann, 1989)
- Poor memory (Ewing-Cobbs, Fletcher, & Levin, 1985; Pang, 1985; Szekeres, Ylvisaker, & Holland, 1985)
- Reduced orientation (Haarbauer-Krupa, Moser, Smith, Sullivan, & Szekeres, 1985)
- Reduced attention (Adamovich, Henderson, & Auerbach, 1985; Szekeres et al., 1985)
- Impulsivity (Ylvisaker & Weinstein, 1989)
- Reduced alertness and awareness (Brink, Imbus, & Woo-San, 1980)
- Confusion
- Reduced visual perception skills (Szekeres et al., 1985)
- Language and cognitive deficits (Ewing-Cobbs et al., 1985)
- Reduced organization, reasoning, problem solving, and judgment skills (Szekeres et al., 1985)
- Emotional lability (Pang, 1985)
- Presence of primitive reflexes (Ylvisaker & Logemann, 1985)
- Abnormal muscle tone (Jaffe, Mastrilli, Molitor, & Valko, 1985; Pang, 1985)

</td><td>

Related Feeding Characteristics

- Slow initiation of voluntary movement, including mouth opening and posterior propulsion of the bolus (Logemann, 1989)
- Immature feeding and swallowing patterns (Ylvisaker & Logemann, 1985)
- Oral hypersensitivity
- Bite reflex
- Absent or delayed initiation of pharyngeal swallow (Lazarus & Logemann, 1987; Ylvisaker & Logemann, 1985; Ylvisaker & Weinstein, 1989)

</td></tr>
</table>

Prematurity of Birth/Low Birth Weight

The following characteristics vary depending on the degree of prematurity, as well as presence of other medical complications. As previously noted in the *Normal Oral-Motor and Swallowing Development* section, sucking does not mature until 30 to 34 weeks gestation. Frequent complications associated with prematurity include poor lung development; frequent respiratory distress (Babson, Gorham, & Benson, 1966); intracranial birth injuries secondary to traumatic birth, anoxia, and subarachnoid and intraventricular hemorrhages; neonatal infections; congenital malformations, such as tracheoesophageal fistula (Babson et al., 1966; Hill, 1975); atresia of the digestive tract; and diaphragmatic hernia (Hill, 1975). Low-birth-weight babies are more likely to suffer from congenital malformations (Hill, 1975).

General Characteristics

- Low birth weight (Hill, 1975)
- Hydrocephalus (McCormick, 1989)
- Cerebral palsy (Babson et al., 1966; McCormick, 1989)
- Seizure disorder (McCormick, 1989)
- Sensorineural impairment (McCormick, 1989)
- Developmental delay (McCormick, 1989)
- Low Apgar scores (McCormick, 1989)
- Cardiac failure (Babson et al., 1966)
- Hyperirritability (Babson et al., 1966)
- Lethargy (Babson et al., 1966)
- Hypotonia (Babson et al., 1966)
- Increased or decreased head growth (Babson et al., 1966)
- Bowel obstruction (Babson et al., 1966)
- Strabismus and retrolental fibroplasia (Babson et al., 1966)

Related Feeding Characteristics

- Intrauterine aspiration (Babson et al., 1966)
- Hypersensitivity
- Difficulty coordinating sucking and breathing (Morris, 1989)
- Hyperextension of head/neck secondary to positioning in the Neonatal Intensive Care Unit to increase the diameter of the pharynx for more efficient respiration (Morris, 1989)
- Increased incidence of apnea and bradycardia secondary to feeding problems (Mathew, 1988)
- Poor tolerance for fat in cow's milk (Hill, 1975)

Anoxia, Meningitis, and Encephalitis

Lack of blood flow to the brain may result in brain damage. **Anoxia/hypoxia** may be caused by a variety of conditions, including

- perinatal trauma
- near-drowning
- cardiac complications

- pulmonary complications
- traumatic brain injury
- aneurism

Swallowing disorders are often secondary to reduced levels of alertness and responsiveness. Concomitant problems related to other facets of the injury may cause more specific feeding and swallowing problems. **Meningitis** is an inflammation of the meninges surrounding the brain and spinal cord, often caused by bacterial, viral, or fungal source. **Encephalitis** is an inflammation of the brain matter generally caused by viral infection, bacterial abscess, or inflammation. The general characteristics of these are similar. Specific feeding and swallowing problems will vary, but most are secondary to behavioral characteristics and general tone abnormalities.

General Characteristics

- Increased agitation
- Decreased cognition
- Abnormal tone

Related Feeding Characteristics

- Weak suck
- Poor coordination of breathing and swallowing
- Delayed or absent initiation of the pharyngeal swallow

Brain Tumor

Swallowing problems are rarely a predominant characteristic of children who have brain tumors. However, swallowing problems may develop secondary to displacement of the pharyngeal and laryngeal structures, pressure on the brain stem associated with size and location of the tumor, or as a result of the radiation process sometimes used in treatment (Ravindarnath & Cushing, 1982). Gliomas are the most frequently occurring type of brain tumor in children. Medulloblastomas are the second most commonly occurring (Finlay, 1986). Brain stem gliomas are also seen in children. Children with brain stem gliomas are more likely to have oral motor or swallowing problems than children with other types of tumors (Frank, Schwartz, Epstein, & Beresford, 1989).

General Characteristics

- Hypersensitivity secondary to radiation
- Increased agitation
- Cerebellar mutism
- Ataxia (Albright, Price, & Guthkelch, 1983; Frank et al., 1989)
- Diplopia (Albright et al., 1983)
- Headache (Albright et al., 1983)
- Multiple cranial nerve palsies (Albright et al., 1983)

Related Feeding Characteristics

- Changes in taste sensation
- Oral hypersensitivity
- Poor suck response in infants secondary to cranial nerve involvement (Albright et al., 1983)
- Delay in the pharyngeal swallow
- Backflow secondary to decreased tone in lower esophageal sphincter (Frank et al., 1989)

Brain Tumor (continued)

General Characteristics

- Vertigo (Albright et al., 1983)
- Irritability and lethargy (Frank et al., 1989)

Related Feeding Characteristics

- Dysarthria
- Vomiting (Albright et al., 1983)
- Possible reduced salivary gland function

Children with HIV/AIDS

The greatest percent of infants with human immunodeficiency virus (HIV) are infected *in vitro* from HIV-positive or acquired immune deficiency syndrome (AIDS)-infected mothers (Pressman & Morrison, 1988). The incidence of AIDS is expected to rise as a leading cause of death as more infants are born to HIV-positive women (*Early Intervention Quarterly Newsletter,* 1989). Children who display symptoms before 24 months of age have poor outcome, with many dying within 12 months of diagnosis (*Early Intervention Quarterly Newsletter,* 1989). Medical complications are numerous and include brain tumors and encephalopathy, which, in turn, lead to severe dysphagia (Pressman & Morrison, 1988).

General Characteristics

- Bacterial and lung infections (*Early Intervention Quarterly Newsletter,* 1989)
- Developmental delays (*Early Intervention Quarterly Newsletter,* 1989; Pressman & Morrison, 1988)
- Failure to thrive (Pressman & Morrison, 1988)
- Progressive neurologic deterioration (Pressman & Morrison, 1988)
- Hypoxia (Pressman & Morrison, 1988)
- Cardiomyopathy (Pressman & Morrison, 1988)

Related Feeding Characteristics

- Pain with swallowing/odynophagia (Pressman & Morrison, 1988)
- Malnutrition leading to muscle wasting (Pressman & Morrison, 1988)
- Poor appetite (Pressman & Morrison, 1988)
- Dysphagia secondary to thrush and candida (Pressman & Morrison, 1988)
- Poor dentition (Pressman & Morrison, 1988)

Children Born to Cocaine-Dependent Mothers

Use of cocaine by a pregnant woman may result in neurologic damage, medical complications, and physical abnormalities in the developing fetus. Postnatally, poor maternal bonding, inadequate nutrition, and prolonged hospitalization further impede normal development.

Cocaine is not evident in an adult's urine after 24 hours. However, its presence may be noted in a pregnant woman's urine and the urine of a newborn for 4 to 7 days (Bingol et al., 1987; Chasnoff, 1987).

General Characteristics	*Related Feeding Characteristics*
• Increased agitation	• Feeding intolerance (Cherukuri et al., 1988)
• Irritability (Chasnoff, Burns, & Burns, 1987)	• Poor coordination of suck and swallow (Lewis, Bennett, & Schmeder, 1989)
• Lower Apgar scores (MacGregor et al., 1987)	• Inability to stabilize tongue in midline (Lewis et al., 1989)
• Lower birth weight (MacGregor et al., 1987)	• Tremors in tongue (Lewis et al., 1989)
• Small for gestational age (MacGregor et al., 1987)	

Children with Down Syndrome

Most children who have Down syndrome present with global developmental delays. Accordingly, feeding and swallowing skills also develop at a later date (Pueschel, 1984). There are three phenotypes associated with Down syndrome: trisomy 21, translocation, or mosaicism. Trisomy 21 is most common, accounting for 95 percent of individuals with Down syndrome (Jung, 1989).

General Characteristics	*Related Feeding Characteristics*
• General developmental delay	• Increased drooling (Palmer & Ekvall, 1978)
• Hypotonia	• Tongue protrusion (Palmer & Ekvall, 1978)
• Hearing loss (Jung, 1989)	• Poor sucking and swallowing (Calvert, Vivian, & Calvert, 1976; Palmer & Ekvall, 1978)
• Delayed tooth eruption (Jung, 1989)	• Reduced chewing (Calvert et al., 1976; Palmer & Ekvall, 1978)
	• Shortened buccal cavity (Stoel-Gammon, 1982)
	• Small oral cavity (Stoel-Gammon, 1981)
	• High palate (Stoel-Gammon, 1981)
	• Obstruction of nasal passages (Stoel-Gammon, 1981)
	• Velopharyngeal dysfunction (Jung, 1989)
	• Small mandible (Ardran, Marker, & Kemp, 1972)
	• Abnormal dental bite (Jung, 1989)
	• Unusually high pharynx (Stoel-Gammon, 1981)

Stroke

Strokes in childhood are primarily seen in children with sickle cell disease (Powers, Wilson, Imbus, Pegelow, & Allen, 1978) but also may be secondary to congenital malformations or may accompany syndromes such as Moya Moya (Rogers & Coleman, 1992; Takashita, Kagawa, Izawa, & Kitamura, 1986). In one study, 46.2 percent of juvenile hemorrhagic strokes were caused by primary hemorrhage, 38.5 percent were due to arteriovenous malformations, 5.7 percent were related to intracranial aneurysm, and Moya Moya syndrome accounted for 5.7 percent (Takashita et al., 1986).

Characteristics will vary according to site and size of lesion, developmental level at the time of stroke, and history of strokes. Some of the deficits are directly related to the site of lesion. Other behaviors/patterns are secondary factors that interfere. There is limited research regarding disorders of feeding and swallowing with children who have had strokes.

General Characteristics

- Possible hemiplegia
- Seizure disorder (Powers et al., 1978)
- Cognitive deficits
- Language deficits

Related Feeding Characteristics

- Unilateral or bilateral facial weakness
- Unilateral or bilateral oral/motor dysfunction possibly impeding labial and lingual movement
- Loss of liquid/food
- Decreased tongue lateralization
- Decreased bolus formation
- Decreased bolus manipulation
- Decreased rotary chew
- Delay in pharyngeal swallow

SUMMARY

Before evaluating an infant or child, it is essential for the clinician to have a thorough understanding of the normal developmental process. Equally important is basic knowledge regarding developmental and acquired disorders and potential related feeding and swallowing problems.

Chapter 4 presents a feeding and swallowing assessment procedure that provides a thorough, yet efficient tool for evaluating feeding and swallowing problems. The tool was designed for clinicians with all levels of experience in a variety of settings including hospitals, schools, and clinics. It may be used by the experienced clinician to record evaluation results or by the new clinician as a step-by-step guide through the assessment.

REFERENCES

Adamovich, B., Henderson, J., & Auerbach, S. (1985). *Cognitive rehabilitation of closed head injured patients: A dynamic approach.* Boston: College-Hill Press.

Albright, L., Price, R., & Guthkelch, N. (1983). Brain stem gliomas in children. *Cancer, 52*, 2313–2319.

Alexander, R. (1988). *Early feeding, sound production, and pre-linguistic/cognitive development and their relationship to gross-motor and fine-motor development.* Paper presented at The Rehabilitation Institute of Chicago, Chicago, Illinois.

Ardran, G., Harker, P., & Kemp, P. (1972). Tongue size in Down syndrome. *Journal of Mental Deficiency Research, 16*, 160–166.

Babson, S., Gorham, R., & Benson, R. (1966). *Primer on prematurity and high risk pregnancy.* St. Louis: C.V. Mosby.

Bailey, D., & Wolery, M. (1989). *Assessing infants and preschoolers with handicaps.* Columbus, OH: Merrill.

Bingol, N., Fuchs, M., Diaz, V., Stone, R., & Gromisch, D. (1987). Teratogenicity of cocaine in humans. *Journal of Pediatrics, 110*, 93–96.

Bosma, J.F. (1978). Structure and function of the infant oral and pharyngeal mechanisms. In J. Wilson (Ed.), *Oral-motor function and dysfunction in children* (pp. 33–65). Chapel Hill, NC: University of North Carolina Press.

Brink, J., Imbus, C., & Woo-San, J. (1980). Physical recovery after severe closed head injury in children and adolescents. *Journal of Pediatrics, 97* (5), 721–727.

Bu'Lock, F., Woolridge, M., & Baum, J. (1990). Development of co-ordination of sucking, swallowing and breathing: Ultrasound study of term and preterm infants. *Developmental Medicine and Child Neurology, 32*, 669–678.

Calvert, S., Vivian, V., & Calvert, G. (1976). Dietary adequacy, feeding practices, and feeding behavior of children with Down's syndrome. *Journal of American Dietetic Association, 69*, 152–156.

Chasnoff, I. (1987). Perinatal effects of cocaine. *Contemporary Obstetrics and Gynecology, 29*, 163–179.

Chasnoff, I., Burns, K., & Burns, W. (1987). Cocaine use in pregnancy: Perinatal morbidity and mortality. *Neurotoxicology and Teratology, 9*, 241–243.

Cherukuri, R., Minkoff, J., Feldman, J., Parekh, A., & Glass, L. (1988). A cohort study of alkaloidil cocaine ("crack") in pregnancy. *Obstetrics and Gynecology, 72*, 147–151.

Committee on Nutrition, American Academy of Pediatrics. (1985). *Pediatric nutrition handbook.* In G.B. Forbes & C. Woodruf (Eds.). Elk Grove Village, IL: American Academy of Pediatrics.

Connor, F., Williamson, G., & Siepp, J. (Eds.). (1978). *Program guide for infants and toddlers with neuromotor and other developmental disabilities.* New York: Teachers' College Press.

Early Intervention Quarterly Newsletter of the Illinois Birth to Three Clearinghouse. (1989). *Pediatric aids: Facts and family needs, 4* (1), 1–3.

Ewing-Cobbs, L., Fletcher, J., & Levin, H. (1985). Neuropsychological sequelae following pediatric head injury. In M. Ylvisaker (Ed.), *Head injury rehabilitation: Children and adolescents* (pp. 71–90). Boston: College-Hill Press.

Finlay, J.L. (1986). Natural history and epidemiology of medulloblastoma. In P.M. Zeltzer & C. Pochedly (Eds.), *Medulloblastomas in children: New concepts in tumor biology, diagnosis, and treatment* (pp. 22–36). New York: Prager.

Frank, Y., Schwartz, S., Epstein, N., & Beresford, H. (1989). Chronic dysphagia, vomiting and gastroesophageal reflux as manifestations of a brainstem glioma: A case study. *Pediatric Neuroscience, 15* (5), 265–268.

Grand, R., Watkins, J., & Torti, F. (1976). Development of the human gastro intestinal tract. *Gastroenterology, 70* (2), 790–810.

Griggs, C., Jones, P., & Lee, R. (1989). Videofluoroscopic investigation of feeding disorders of children with multiple handicaps. *Developmental Medicine and Child Neurology, 31* (3), 303–308.

Haarbauer-Krupa, J., Moser, L., Smith, G., Sullivan, D., & Szekeres, S. (1985). Cognitive rehabilitation therapy: Middle stages of recovery. In M. Ylvisaker (Ed.), *Head injury rehabilitation: Children and adolescents* (pp. 287–310). Boston: College-Hill Press.

Helfrich-Miller, K., Rector, K., & Straka, J. (1986). Dysphagia: Its treatment in the profoundly retarded patient with cerebral palsy. *Archives of Physical Medicine and Rehabilitation, 67* (8), 520–525.

Hill, E. (1975). *The preterm baby and other babies with low birth weight.* New York: Churchill Livingstone.

Jaffe, M., Mastrilli, J., Molitor, C., & Valko, A. (1985). Intervention for motor disorders. In M. Ylvisaker (Ed.), *Head injury rehabilitation: Children and adolescents* (pp.167–194). Boston: College-Hill Press.

Jones, P. (1989). Feeding disorders in children with multiple handicaps. *Developmental Medicine and Child Neurology, 31* (3), 404–406.

Jung, J. (1989). *Genetic syndromes in communication disorders.* Boston: College-Hill Press.

Kramer, S. (1985). Special swallowing problems in children. *Gastrointestinal Radiology, 10,* 241–250.

Lazarus, C., & Logemann, J. (1987). Swallowing disorders in closed head trauma patients. *Archives of Physical Medicine and Rehabilitation, 68,* 79–84.

Levitt, S. (1982). *Treatment of cerebral palsy and motor delay.* Oxford, England: Blackwell Scientific Publications.

Lewis, K., Bennett, B., & Schmeder, N. (1989). The care of infants menaced by cocaine abuse. *Maternal and Child Nutrition, 14,* 324–329.

Logemann, J. (1983). *Evaluation and treatment of swallowing disorders.* San Diego, CA: College-Hill Press.

Logemann, J. (1989). Evaluation and treatment planning for the head-injured patient with oral intake disorders. *Journal of Head Trauma Rehabilitation, 4* (4), 24–33.

Logemann, J. (1990). *Infant swallowing.* Miniseminar presented at the meeting of the Illinois Speech-Language-Hearing Association, Chicago, Illinois.

MacGregor, S., Keith, L., Chasnoff, I., Rosner, M., Chisum, G., Shaw, P., & Minoque, J. (1987). Cocaine use during pregnancy: Adverse perinatal outcome. *American Journal of Obstetrics and Gynecology, 157,* 686–690.

Mathew, O.P. (1988). Respiratory control during nipple feeding in preterm infants. *Pediatric Pulmonology, 5* (4), 220–224.

McCormick, M. (1989). Long-term follow-up of infants discharged from neonatal intensive care units. *Journal of the American Medical Association, 261* (12), 1767–1772.

McGee, M. (1987). *Neurodevelopmental treatment: Pediatric certification course.* Winston-Salem, North Carolina.

Morris, S. (1989). Development of oral-motor skills in the neurologically impaired child receiving non-oral feedings. *Dysphagia, 3,* 135–154.

Morris, S., & Klein, M. (1987). *Pre-feeding skills.* Tucson, AZ: Therapy Skill Builders.

Palmer, S., & Ekvall, S. (1978). *Pediatric nutrition in developmental disorders.* Springfield, IL: Charles C Thomas.

Pang, D. (1985). Pathophysiologic correlates of neurobehavioral syndromes following closed head injury. In M. Ylvisaker (Ed.), *Head injury rehabilitation: Children and adolescents* (pp. 3–70). Boston: College-Hill Press.

Powers, D., Wilson, B., Imbus, C., Pegelow, C., & Allen, J. (1978). The natural history of stroke in sickle cell disease. *The American Journal of Medicine, 65,* 461–470.

Pressman, H., & Morrison, S. (1988). Dysphagia in the pediatric AIDS population. *Dysphagia, 2,* 166–169.

Pritchard, J. (1966). Fetal swallowing and amniotic fluid volume. *Obstetrics and Gynecology, 28* (5), 607–610.

Pueschel, S. (1984). *The young child with Down syndrome.* New York: Human Sciences Press.

Ravindarnath, Y., & Cushing, B. (1982). Neuroblastoma of the neck and chest. In C. Pochedly (Ed.), *Neuroblastoma: Clinical and biological manifestations* (pp. 39–49). New York: Elsevier Biomedical.

Rogers, P., & Coleman, M. (1992). *Medical care in Down syndrome: A preventive medicine approach.* New York: Marcel Dekker.

Rossetti, L. (1990). *The Rosetti infant-toddler language scale.* East Moline, IL: Linguisystems.

Stoel-Gammon, C. (1981). Speech development of infants and children with Down syndrome. In J. Darby, Jr. (Ed.), *Speech evaluation in medicine* (pp. 341–360). New York: Grune & Stratton.

Szekeres, S., Ylvisaker, M., & Holland, A. (1985). Cognitive rehabilitation therapy: A framework for intervention. In M. Ylvisaker (Ed.), *Head injury rehabilitation: Children and adolescents* (pp. 219–246). Boston: College-Hill Press.

Takashita, M., Kagawa, M., Izawa, M., & Kitamura, K. (1986). Hemorrhagic stroke in infancy, childhood and adolescence. *Surgical Neurology, 26,* 496–500.

Tuchman, D. (1988). Dysfunctional swallowing in the pediatric patient: Clinical considerations. *Dysphagia, 2,* 203–208.

Tuchman, D. (1989). Cough, choke, sputter: The evaluation of the child with dysfunctional swallowing. *Dysphagia, 3,* 111–116.

Weiss, M. (1988). Dysphagia in infants and children. *Otolaryngologic Clinics of North America, 21* (4), 727–735.

Ylvisaker, M., & Logemann, J. (1985). Therapy for feeding and swallowing disorders following head injury. In M. Ylvisaker (Ed.), *Head injury rehabilitation; Children and adolescents* (pp. 195–215). Boston: College-Hill Press.

Ylvisaker, M., & Weinstein, M. (1989). Recovery of oral feeding after pediatric head injury. *Journal of Head Trauma Rehabilitation, 4* (4), 51–63.

◆ CHAPTER 3 ◆

Clinical Evaluation of Dysphagia in Adults

Leora R. Cherney, Jean J. Pannell, and Carol A. Cantieri

A comprehensive evaluation of the patient's swallowing mechanism is a multistep process which may include the following:

- prefeeding assessment including a complete history of the problem and observation of oral, pharyngeal, and laryngeal structures and function
- clinical evaluation of swallowing
- radiographic assessment of the swallowing mechanism or use of other instrumental procedures

This process, which may be modified according to the needs and circumstances of each individual patient, enables the clinician to gain maximum information about all physiologic phases of swallowing as well as to observe the patient's actual performance in a functional setting. In this chapter, guidelines for the prefeeding assessment and the clinical evaluation of swallowing are described. A series of forms for documenting the results of the prefeeding assessment and the clinical evaluation are presented. Also, ways of disseminating evaluation results to team members, patients, and families are described.

EVALUATION OF PREFEEDING SKILLS

Before the oral intake of any food substances, important medical and safety information is obtained from the patient, caregiver, or physician or from the patient's medical chart. Additional information is obtained by observing the patient and from an oral-pharyngeal sensorimotor evaluation. At the completion of the preassessment, the clinician should be able to make preliminary decisions

49

regarding potential for oral intake and the need for further evaluation procedures and referrals.

A prefeeding evaluation form has been devised to guide the clinician in the collection and documentation of relevant information. The prefeeding evaluation is typically completed for those patients who are potentially at high risk for aspiration (e.g., those patients who are not yet eating orally or those with tracheostomies). The form also may be used for screening oral, pharyngeal, and laryngeal functioning before the administration of the clinical evaluation of swallowing.

An alternate preassessment form is included in Chapter 4. Although this form was designed primarily for the pediatric patient, it also may be appropriate for the adult patient.

Medical/Nutritional Status

Check the patient's medical status for significant information regarding swallowing and nutritional status. This might include coexisting medical problems such as

- chronic obstructive pulmonary disease
- prior surgeries involving the head and neck area or the gastrointestinal tract
- current and past medications that might affect swallowing (Stoschus & Allescher, 1993)

Note the duration and frequency of any subjective complaints of swallowing difficulty (Hendrix, 1993). Symptoms such as weight loss, appetite changes, dry mouth, mouth or throat pain, heartburn, regurgitation, and voice changes may be indicative of a swallowing problem.

Respiratory Status

There is a close relationship between the pulmonary mechanism and swallowing function. Indicate whether respiratory rate is within the normal adult ranges of 12 to 16 breaths per minute (Perlman et al., 1991). Note the presence of respiratory symptoms that may be related to the presence of a dysphagia, such as chronic coughing, shortness of breath, and asthmatic episodes.

History of Aspiration

Indicate whether the patient has a history of aspiration pneumonia. This is usually indicative of a dysphagia.

Tracheostomy

If the patient has a tracheostomy, note the type and size. If a cuff is present, record whether it is inflated, partially inflated, or deflated. Make sure that this is in accordance with the physician's orders. If suctioning is required, indicate the frequency. Note any other information related to the tracheostomy such as the consistency and color of the secretions or whether there is a corking schedule.

Level of Responsiveness

Observe and record the patient's general level of alertness, including his or her ability to follow verbal commands.

Behavioral Characteristics

Note the presence of agitation, disorientation, impulsivity, or other behavioral characteristics that could affect his or her attention to the feeding process.

Current Feeding Methods

Indicate whether food intake is oral. If an alternate feeding method is required, document the type [e.g., nasogastric (NG) tube, surgically placed gastrostomy tube (G-tube), percutaneous endoscopic gastrostomy (PEG)] and when it was placed. Note the frequency and amount of food intake, and any other information relevant to the patient's method of food intake.

Positioning

Observe and record the patient's habitual body position, muscle tone, head and neck position, and motor control. Indicate the presence of any interfering patterns such as abnormal reflexes or compensatory motor behaviors.

Determine the best possible position for feeding and document this position on the form. Positioning is important even though food is not administered, because the prefeeding evaluation includes observing the patient handling his or her own secretions and the stimulation of a swallow. The optimal starting position is generally upright at 90 degrees, with the head tilted slightly forward. This position achieves maximum protection of the airway and reduces the chance of aspiration. The weaker side should be supported so that it is elevated above the stronger side. This allows greater control because the food is more likely to fall to the stronger side.

In general, the patient should be supported in a relaxed position to reduce excessive muscle tone and extraneous head and body movements. This reduces any internal distractions from body pain or discomfort and enables the patient to attend more fully during the evaluation. Often raising the back of the bed and using physical supports such as pillows and wedges is helpful. In cases in which the patient is unable to achieve optimal positioning, consultation with physical therapists, occupational therapists, or nursing may be indicated.

Observation of Oral Motor, Pharyngeal, and Laryngeal Functioning

These observations are made without ingestion of any food substances. Results of these observations can help determine whether the patient is an appropriate candidate for further evaluation of oral feeding and swallowing.

Observe the lips, tongue, and mandible at rest. Note their general structure, symmetry, habitual position at rest, and the presence of involuntary movements. Note the presence of any drooling. Observe the status of the oral mucosa (e.g., moistness) and the condition of the patient's dentition.

Record if the patient can produce phonation, and note the quality and strength of his or her voice. This provides an estimate of the patient's ability to achieve laryngeal closure and to protect the airway. A hoarse voice quality may indicate reduced laryngeal closure. A wet or gurgly vocal quality may indicate pooling of saliva or secretions at the laryngeal level. Listen to the patient's speech because the precision and speed of the patient's articulation may provide information about the integrity of the oral motor system that is also involved in swallowing. The presence of hyper- or hyponasality may be indicative of velopharyngeal problems.

Cough

Determine the presence or absence of a voluntary cough and note its strength. If an involuntary cough is observed during the evaluation, document it on the form. This provides an estimate of the patient's ability to achieve laryngeal closure and to protect the airway.

Gag Reflex

Attempt to elicit a gag reflex by stimulating the base of the tongue or the posterior pharyngeal wall with the head of a laryngeal mirror. Compare and record the strength of the reflex after stimulation to both sides. Although a diminished or absent gag does not necessarily indicate swallowing difficulty, it may provide some information about both cranial nerve dysfunction and airway protection.

Voluntary Swallow

Ask the patient to swallow, and document if he or she can perform a dry swallow on command. Note and record the presence or absence of laryngeal elevation, which may indicate that a swallow has occurred. If this is difficult to observe, place your hand on the throat at the level of the larynx to feel this movement. Logemann (1983) suggested the following technique to estimate oropharyngeal transit time:

> The index finger should be positioned immediately behind the mandible anteriorly, the middle finger at the hyoid bone, the third finger at the top of the thyroid cartilage, and the fourth finger at the bottom of the thyroid cartilage. As the patient swallows, the clinician's fingers on the patient's neck can assess initiation of tongue movement on the basis of movement felt by the index finger at the submandibular area immediately behind the anterior mandible. The second finger can perceive hyoid bone movement, and the third and fourth fingers can define laryngeal movement when the swallowing reflex triggers. Com-

paring the time elapsed between initiation of tongue movement and initiation of hyoid and laryngeal movement can provide the clinician with a very rough estimate of oral transit time, or the time taken from initiation of the swallow by the tongue until the swallowing reflex triggers. (p.120)

Other Observations

Record additional pertinent information such as drooling, mouth odor, and abnormal reflexes affecting feeding (e.g., tonic bite reflex, tongue thrust).

Response to Stimulation

Observe the patient's responsiveness to stimulation, noting the adequacy of lip closure or protrusion, the presence of a bite reflex, and the presence of a pharyngeal swallow. Stimulation may be applied as follows:

1. Apply pressure to the lips and tongue with a tongue depressor or your fingers. Be cautious if the patient has a bite reflex. Note the tone and differential response to light and firm touch. Also note the presence of lip closure and/or protrusion.
2. Place an empty spoon into the patient's mouth to stimulate a dry swallow. Pressure to the anterior third of the tongue may facilitate this response.
3. Rub the lips, teeth, gums, and tongue with a lemon glycerin swab that has been almost entirely squeezed out. This may aid in stimulating the pharyngeal swallow and provide some indication of the patient's responsiveness to taste.
4. Provide thermal stimulation by tapping the base of the anterior faucial pillars several times with an ice-cold small metal spoon or a laryngoscopic mirror (size 00) to facilitate a pharyngeal swallow. It may be necessary to verbally request the patient to swallow after stimulation.

Recommendations

Determine the appropriate plan of action. The following signs may indicate that the patient is at high risk for aspiration and should remain prohibited from oral intake (NPO):

- reduced alertness
- reduced responsiveness to stimulation
- absent swallow
- absent protective cough
- difficulty handling secretions as evidenced by excessive coughing and choking, copious secretions, and a wet gurgly voice quality
- significant reductions in the range and strength of oral, pharyngeal, and laryngeal movements

For those patients who exhibit some alertness and responsiveness to stimulation yet remain at high risk for aspiration, a videofluoroscopic examination is typically recommended before the clinical evaluation. For most other patients, videofluoroscopy is indicated after the clinical evaluation.

An otolaryngology (ENT) consult for laryngeal endoscopy may be indicated for those patients exhibiting any difficulty at the laryngeal level, especially those with a weak or absent cough and/or breathy or hoarse vocal quality. Document any other recommendations, including the need for other diagnostic imaging techniques or referral to a gastroenterologist to evaluate swallow dysfunction in the esophageal phase.

Goals

Although a patient may remain NPO, treatment may be recommended to improve prefeeding skills such as oral-pharyngeal sensorimotor functioning or alertness and responsiveness. Treatment goals can be documented on the prefeeding form. If, however, treatment is deferred for any reason (e.g., pending the results of further evaluations), note this on the form.

Patient/Family Counseling

Document any patient and family counseling. Note whether the patient and family are in agreement with the goals delineated above.

CLINICAL EVALUATION OF DYSPHAGIA

The clinical evaluation is an "indispensable part of the overall evaluation of dysphagia" (Miller, 1984) because of the practical and functional data gained. This examination is useful in identifying the area(s) of dysfunction and in recognizing patients at risk for aspiration who require further evaluation (Linden & Siebens, 1983; Logemann, 1983). It allows for the assessment of behaviors that may interfere with, or compensate for, the patient's swallowing skills (e.g., rate and quantity of intake, and general level of awareness) (Leopold & Kagel, 1983). Also, because the evaluation can be administered promptly on patient referral, it provides immediate information for management and treatment.

In the following section, procedural guidelines are presented for the clinical evaluation of swallowing in those patients whom it is predicted will tolerate at least one food consistency. The procedures used and types of precautions necessary for the clinical evaluation will differ for each patient. However, in general, guidelines can be recommended for each of the following three groups of patients:

- patients whose primary means of nutrition is by an alternate feeding method
- patients with a tracheostomy
- patients who are already receiving an oral diet

Then the Clinical Evaluation of Dysphagia (CED) form is described. This form follows the stages of the normal swallow process (i.e., oral and pharyngeal). The clinician can use this form to document *observable* behaviors during oral intake of six different food consistencies:

- thin liquids
- thick liquids
- pureed foods
- ground solids
- chopped solids
- regular solids

GUIDELINES FOR EVALUATING PATIENTS WITH SEVERE DYSPHAGIA

The following protocols are recommended for those patients whose primary means of nutrition is by an alternate feeding method such as a nasogastric tube or a gastrostomy.

1. Administer the prefeeding evaluation. If the patient has a tracheostomy, refer to the following section for precautions and suggested procedures for evaluating tracheostomy patients.
2. Be sure the patient is in an optimal starting position for feeding (i.e., upright at 90 degrees, head tilted slightly forward, and weaker side elevated above the stronger side).
3. Present the patient with a small ice chip from a spoon. Use of an ice chip is recommended because it is relatively safe if partially aspirated (Miller, 1992). Also, the cold may aid facilitation of the pharyngeal swallow. Observe lip function, tongue propulsion, any chewing ability and the initiation of the pharyngeal swallow. An estimation of oropharyngeal transit time can also be made using the procedure described previously.

   The manner of presentation of the ice chip will vary depending on the patient's lip and tongue function.

   - If lip closure and posterior tongue propulsion are adequate, place the tip of the spoon to the lips and allow the patient to retrieve the ice chip independently from the spoon.
   - If lip closure is reduced but posterior tongue propulsion is adequate, present the ice chip with a spoon. Press down on the anterior third of the tongue, withdrawing the spoon at an upward angle to facilitate lip retrieval of the ice chip from the utensil.
   - If the patient cannot propel the ice chip posteriorly with the tongue, place the ice chip on the back of the tongue.

   If the patient appears to have difficulty with the ice chip, extra caution needs to be taken in completing the evaluation.
4. Because different problems may occur with different food consistencies, assessment for most patients should include a variety of consistencies unless contraindicated because of medical or behavioral problems. Decisions regarding the sequence of presentation of different food consistencies should be based on the patient's history, his or her medical status, prior observations

of the patient, and suspected areas of difficulty. For example, if a delayed pharyngeal swallow is suspected during performance with the ice chip, pureed foods and thick liquids should be presented before thin liquids to reduce the possibility of aspiration. If upper esophageal sphincter dysfunction is suspected from patient complaints of discomfort, thin liquids should be presented first, because this is the easiest consistency for patients with this problem to manage. If possible, observe the patient with small amounts of all the following consistencies for a more comprehensive evaluation (Hutchins & Giancarlo, 1991):

- thin liquids—liquids that are clear with little or no body to them (e.g., water, tea)
- thick liquids—liquids that have body to them (e.g., apricot/peach nectar, creamed soups)
- pureed food—items that are smooth and soft and do not require chewing (e.g., applesauce, whipped potatoes)
- ground solids—items that can be ground (e.g., ground beef, rice)
- chopped solids—items that can be cut to the size of a fingernail or smaller
- regular solids—all types and sizes of food

When presenting liquids or pureed foods, use a spoon. Depending on the degree of lip and tongue movements, use the same presentation procedures as described for the presentation of ice chips. It is safest to begin with small amounts ($^1/_4$ teaspoon). Gradually increase the amounts of each presentation up to 1 to 2 teaspoons of each consistency. Be sure to watch for any signs of difficulty after each presentation such as coughing or choking.

5. Some clinicians place a stethoscope against the patient's neck during the swallow to listen to the occurrence of the swallow and also to detect a characteristic sound that suggests aspiration.
6. Ask the patient to phonate after each swallow, and note any changes in vocal quality (e.g., wet or gurgly), which may indicate pooling at the laryngeal level.
7. Examine the oral cavity for pocketing of food, which may indicate reduced bolus formation and/or sensory loss.
8. If the patient is successful with taking liquids from a spoon, also assess his or her ability to take liquids through a straw or from a cup. Control the amount of liquid by closing the top of the straw with a thumb and allowing the patient to suck from the other end or by limiting the amount of liquid in the cup. Use a cut-out cup to help the patient maintain the optimal tilted-forward head position. These cups are commercially available or can be made by cutting a semicircle out of one side of the rim of a paper cup.
9. Contingent on the patient's success with liquids and pureed foods, present ground or chopped solids. The manner of presentation will vary, depending on the patient's oral-motor functioning. Place a small piece of solid food

- midline on the tongue
- laterally on the good side of the tongue
- between the molars on the good side

If the patient does not voluntarily initiate chewing, rub the lateral side of the tongue with the soft solid to facilitate a chewing response.

10. To reduce the risk of aspiration of any residual food in the oral, velopharyngeal, or pharyngeal areas, seat the patient upright for at least 30 minutes after the clinical evaluation. Monitor the patient for any changes in his or her respiratory or medical status over a 24-hour period (e.g., increased temperature and/or increased amount of secretions).

11. Document all findings on the CED form, as described later in this chapter.

12. For those patients exhibiting some signs of aspiration, a videofluoroscopic evaluation should be completed before starting an oral feeding program. The videofluoroscopic evaluation will help pinpoint the precise area of difficulty and determine if oral feeding is safe at this time. For those patients who exhibit no signs of aspiration, a trial oral feeding program may be initiated. However, a videofluoroscopic evaluation often is recommended to confirm the results of the clinical evaluation and to help determine appropriate compensatory head postures and swallowing techniques that may be necessary for safe swallowing.

GUIDELINES FOR EVALUATING PATIENTS WITH A TRACHEOSTOMY

A tracheostomy tube is placed in those patients who have respiratory difficulties. Such patients are also at greater risk for aspiration. Therefore, special consideration must be given to the evaluation and management of their dysphagia. For clinicians unfamiliar with inflating and deflating cuffed tracheostomies, with suctioning, and with medical emergency techniques, it is recommended that this evaluation be conducted together with nursing or other appropriate medical personnel.

1. Administer the prefeeding evaluation. It is important to know why the tracheostomy was necessary (e.g., airway protection, paralyzed vocal cord, tissue mass, or airway obstruction).

2. Be sure the patient is seated in an optimal position for feeding (i.e., upright at 90 degrees, head tilted slightly forward, and weaker side elevated above the stronger side).

3. If the patient has a cuffed tracheostomy, check with the physician regarding the advisability of cuff deflation. There are several problems that may be created by inflation of the cuff during swallowing. These include

   - increased compression of the bolus material around the cuff into the tracheal area (Johnson & Johnson, 1976)
   - tracheal irritation (Logemann, 1983)
   - restriction of laryngeal elevation (Logemann, 1983)
   - prevention of the exhalation of pulmonary air that normally clears the larynx (Sasaki, 1980)

   Therefore, cuff deflation is usually recommended during the clinical swallowing evaluation. Furthermore, when the cuff is deflated, it is easier to detect immediately any signs of aspiration. However, there will be cases in which the cuff cannot be deflated, such as with ventilator-dependent patients with severe difficulty protecting the airway. Oral feeding may be premature in those patients with medical conditions that require a cuffed tracheostomy tube (Fleming, 1992).

4. If cuff deflation is permitted, have the trachea stoma suctioned, deflate the cuff, then repeat the suctioning to ensure a clear airway before the feeding evaluation.

5. Present the patient with an ice chip as described in the preceding section. Momentarily occlude the tracheostomy with a finger to establish near-normal tracheal pressure while swallowing (Fleming, 1992; Logemann, 1983). Observe the presence or absence of laryngeal elevation. Look for any signs of difficulty, including coughing, a gurgly vocal quality, or respiratory distress. Suction immediately if any difficulty is noted.

6. If the patient is successful with ice chips, select the appropriate food consistency to begin with. Color it with blue food coloring to contrast with other possible secretions, thereby allowing any aspiration to be readily observed. Present the patient with small amounts ($^1/_4$ teaspoon) of the blue-tinged food/liquid. Momentarily occlude the tracheostomy with a finger to establish near-normal tracheal pressure. Observe for laryngeal elevation and for any signs of difficulty including coughing, gurgling, or leakage of blue substance around the tracheostomy site. If difficulty is noted, suction immediately. If not, increase the amount of food or liquid to 1 to 2 teaspoons. Then suction the trachea and examine for evidence of any blue-tinged substance.

7. Before proceeding to a new consistency, suction the patient again. This helps differentiate the specific consistencies with which the patient is having difficulty. However, remember that the blue food coloring that coats the oropharyngeal mucosa may be seen several minutes after the test swallow as small amounts of blue-tinged secretions. This may not necessarily be an indication of impaired swallowing (Cameron, Reynolds, & Zuidema, 1973).

8. If the patient was fed with the cuff inflated, suction the patient at the end of the swallowing evaluation. Then deflate the cuff slowly and suction again. Observe the amount and quality of the secretions. If any traces of food coloring are observed, this would indicate the possibility of aspiration.

9. Leave the patient's cuff as it was found initially (i.e., inflated to the same level or deflated). Clean out the patient's mouth with a lemon glycerin swab or toothette to remove any remaining blue dye.

10. Keep the patient upright for at least a half-hour after the swallowing evaluation and monitor for any changes in medical or respiratory status for 24 hours (e.g., increased temperature and/or increased amount of secretions).

11. Document all findings on the CED form.

12. For those patients exhibiting some signs of aspiration, a videofluoroscopic evaluation is recommended before the initiation of the oral feeding program to pinpoint the precise area of difficulty and to determine if oral feeding is safe at this time. For those patients who exhibit no signs of aspiration, a trial oral feeding program may be initiated. However, a videofluoroscopic evaluation often is recommended to confirm the results of the clinical

evaluation, and to help determine appropriate compensatory head positions and swallowing techniques that may be necessary for safer swallowing.

When interpreting the patient's performance on the clinical evaluation, the clinician should be aware that swallowing problems may be created by the presence of the tracheostomy itself. For instance, the tracheostomy tube can actually affix the larynx anteriorly, thus restricting normal laryngeal elevation and rotation and resulting in reduced glottal closure and increased laryngeal penetration (Arms, Denes, & Tintsman, 1974; Bonanno, 1971). Aspiration may increase when the tracheostomy tube is not occluded (Muz, Muthog, Nelson, & Jones, 1989). Lack of movement of the laryngeal muscles, together with restricted movement of the pretracheal strap muscles, can interfere with the relaxation of the cricopharyngeal sphincter (Bonanno, 1971). Also, the upper airway is occluded, which interferes with the patient's ability to expel air to clear the larynx of foreign material (Sasaki, Suzuki, Horiuchi, & Kurchner, 1977; Weaver & Fleming, 1978). However, Logemann (1983) reported these problems to be generally rare in occurrence and stated that among more than 2,000 patients with swallowing deficits evaluated at Northwestern University, only one had swallowing problems directly attributable to the tracheostomy tube.

There is some controversy regarding the treatment of swallowing in patients with tracheostomy tubes. Some authorities believe that oral intake for either evaluation or treatment purposes should be postponed until the tracheostomy tube is removed. For instance, Bonanno (1971) suggested that oral intake be postponed if the patient's tracheostomy tube is a Jackson size 5 and larger or if the patient is restricted to a cuffed tracheostomy tube. Fleming (1992) also suggested that oral intake be restricted if the patient's respiratory status necessitates an inflated cuff.

In the meantime, treatment goals can be directed toward decannulation. Weaning from the tracheostomy tube can be accomplished by

- gradual reduction in the size of the tracheostomy tube
- removal of the cuff
- introduction of a fenestrated tube
- gradually increasing the period of time that the patient tolerates occlusion, for uncuffed or fenestrated tubes
- use of a one-way Kistner valve that opens on inhalation and closes on exhalation.

In many facilities, swallowing evaluation and treatment may proceed in conjunction with decannulation for those patients who demonstrate limited success with oral intake. The rationale for this is that treatment for swallowing disorders should begin as early as possible. Furthermore, treatment that facilitates the patient's ability to handle his or her secretions may improve candidacy for decannulation.

GUIDELINES FOR EVALUATING PATIENTS RECEIVING AN ORAL DIET

Because patients receiving an oral diet are already experiencing some success with their feeding and swallowing, it is best to observe them at meal time. Look for any indications of difficulty with the different food consistencies such as

- reduced attention and orientation, distractibility
- behaviors, such as impulsivity, affecting rate and amount per mouthful
- abnormal head and body position
- chewing difficulties
- drooling of liquid/bolus
- pocketing
- coughing/choking
- changes in vocal quality
- slow eating

Document all findings on the CED form as described in the following section.

CLINICAL EVALUATION OF DYSPHAGIA: DOCUMENTATION OF RESULTS

The Clinical Evaluation of Dysphagia (CED) form (Appendix 3A) follows the stages of swallowing from the oral phase through the pharyngeal phase. The clinician can use this form to document observable behaviors during oral intake and to infer the underlying deficits contributing to the swallowing dysfunction. Six different food consistencies can be evaluated:

- thin liquids
- thick liquids
- pureed foods
- ground solids
- chopped solids
- regular solids

It is recommended that while you conduct the evaluation, you document your observations and rate performance for each structure and phase. Performance ratings are defined as follows:

- adequate—skills are within normal limits
- adequate but reduced function—patient can consistently perform function, but reductions are evident
- interferes with function—patient can inconsistently perform function
- nonfunctional—patient cannot perform function

General Impressions

Describe briefly the general mealtime environment, including distractions that might adversely affect the patient's attention to the feeding process (Perlman et al., 1991). Also note the patient's positioning, the appearance (e.g., cluttered) and placement of the meal tray, and any important information about what the patient eats and does not eat. For example, some patients may not remove food covers or may not eat any items located on one side of the tray (Perlman et al., 1991). Document any other relevant information.

Oral Phase

Lips

1. Protrusion
   Record whether the patient is able to initiate and maintain protrusion for retrieval from each utensil (i.e., spoon, cup, and straw).
2. Closure
   Record whether the patient can initiate closure for retrieval from the utensil, maintain closure for retrieval from the utensil, or maintain closure throughout the oral stage (i.e., from the presentation of food until the pharyngeal swallow is triggered). Indicate if leakage is observed, and specify the location. If the patient is assessed with a variety of utensils and different food consistencies, record in the appropriate boxes.
3. Interpretation of lip function
   For each consistency, rate the patient's lip function as

   - adequate
   - adequate but reduced
   - interferes with function
   - nonfunctional

Several reasons could account for reductions in function. Record those that appear to be contributing to the problem. These may include

- reduced or increased labial tone
- reduced sensation
- reduced strength
- reduced range of motion
- reduced rate
- inaccurate direction of labial movement

If any abnormal lip reflexes are observed, record them under "Other."

Tongue

1. Bolus formation and transport
   For each food consistency, rate the patient's ability to form and propel the bolus posteriorly as

   - adequate
   - adequate but reduced

- interferes with function
- nonfunctional

Indicate if tongue pumping or a tongue thrust is observed.

2. Food remaining in mouth

If food is observed to remain in the mouth, indicate the location. Note if the patient is aware of this and if the patient can independently clear his or her oral cavity.

3. Cough reflex before swallow

Record whether an early reflexive cough is observed before the pharyngeal swallow for each food consistency. This may be indicative of reduced ability to hold the bolus with the tongue.

4. Interpretation of tongue function

For each food consistency, rate tongue function as

- adequate
- adequate but reduced
- interferes with function
- nonfunctional

Indicate the underlying causes of difficulty. These may include

- reduced or increased lingual tone
- reduced range of motion
- reduced rate
- reduced sensation
- reduced strength
- inaccurate direction of lingual movement

If any abnormal reflexes are observed, record them under "Other."

Mandible

1. Chewing

Record whether the patient chews with a rotary pattern or a vertical chop, or whether chewing is absent.

2. Interpretation of mandibular function

Record interpretations as

- adequate
- adequate but reduced
- interferes with function
- nonfunctional

Indicate underlying causes of difficulty, which may include

- reduced or increased buccal and mandibular tone

- reduced strength
- reduced range of motion
- reduced rate of mandibular movement
- poor or absent dentition
- malocclusion

If any abnormal reflexes are observed, record them under "Other."

Summary: Overall Oral Phase

1. For each consistency, rate the overall oral phase as

   - adequate
   - adequate but reduced
   - interferes with function
   - nonfunctional

2. Summarize and document the main underlying causes of the difficulty. Include any additional comments related to medical or behavioral status that appear to affect the oral stage of the feeding process (e.g., distractibility, perseveration, or fatigue).

Pharyngeal Phase

Although the pharyngeal phase cannot be observed directly without videofluoroscopy, certain behavioral characteristics are indicative of possible deficits in this area. If pharyngeal phase problems are suspected, a videofluoroscopic examination should be completed.

1. Document if the gag reflex and volitional cough are present, diminished, or absent. Although a diminished or absent gag or cough do not necessarily indicate swallowing difficulty, they may provide some information about cranial nerve dysfunction and the ability to achieve laryngeal closure and to protect the airway.

2. For each food consistency, document if there is a cough reflex before the swallow. This may indicate a delayed pharyngeal swallow.

3. Document any observable nasal regurgitation and the consistencies with which it occurs. Nasal regurgitation may be indicative of reduced velopharyngeal closure caused by structural or functional abnormalities.

4. Record whether elevation of the hyoid and thyroid cartilages is observed for each consistency. This usually indicates that the pharyngeal swallow has been initiated, and the larynx has elevated to protect the airway.

5. Indicate whether the initiation of the pharyngeal swallow is delayed and the approximate length of the delay in seconds. Remember that this time passage from the initiation of lingual movement after bolus formation to elevation of the larynx, indicating triggering of the pharyngeal swallow should be approximately 1 second.

6. Record whether repeated swallows are observed for each food presentation, and note the average number required per bolus. Repeated swallows may indicate possible pooling in the pharyngeal area and/or reduced pharyngeal peristalsis.

7. If the patient complains of discomfort during swallowing, record this and have the patient specify the location.

8. Note whether a cough reflex is present either during or after the swallow. A cough reflex during the swallow may indicate reduced vocal cord closure. A cough reflex after the pharyngeal swallow may be indicative of decreased laryngeal elevation, reduced pharyngeal peristalsis, and/or upper esophageal sphincter deficits. Remember that it cannot be assumed that the swallowing process is normal if a cough reflex is not noted, because some patients may not have this protective mechanism. Therefore, videofluoroscopy is always recommended for a complete evaluation of the pharyngeal phase of the swallow.

9. Record any changes in vocal quality after the swallow.

10. Note whether excessive secretions are present.

11. If no difficulties are noted for any consistencies, check "No Problems Exhibited."

Summary: Overall Pharyngeal Phase

1. For each consistency, rate the overall pharyngeal phase as

   • adequate
   • adequate but reduced
   • interferes with function
   • nonfunctional

2. Summarize and document the main underlying causes of the difficulty. Include any additional comments related to medical or behavioral status that affect this stage of the feeding process.

3. Indicate whether the patient appears able or unable to protect his or her airway. This decision should be based on the observations made during the pharyngeal phase (e.g., presence of a cough reflex, and the vocal quality).

Additional Test Results

Document if the patient has been referred for any additional tests such as videofluoroscopy or laryngeal endoscopy. Fill in the results when these tests have been completed. Chapter 5 discusses further the radiographic assessment of dysphagia and provides a model for differential diagnosis based on instrumental techniques.

Severity Level and Neuromuscular Characteristics

On the basis of all the above information, determine the severity level and summarize the predominant characteristics of the dysphagia.

DETERMINING FUNCTIONAL SEVERITY LEVELS FOR DYSPHAGIA AND SETTING GOALS

Exhibit 3-1 is a 7-point severity scale designed to rate the patient's everyday feeding abilities (Steefel, 1981). The items in parentheses indicate suggested associations between the functional severity and the 4-point neuromuscular rating scale on the CED form.

The functional severity level scale for dysphagia provides the basis for developing functional long-term goals. Several factors regarding the patient's projected level of functioning should be considered. These include

- feeding method (oral versus alternate)
- food consistency
- food quantity
- amount of supervision

Following are examples of long-term goals derived from the functional severity level scale.

- consistent oral ingestion, three times daily, of 1 cup of pureed food, presented by nursing staff or family, using prescribed feeding techniques
- consistent oral ingestion of a pureed diet that meets daily nutritional needs, with constant supervision by family
- independent self-feeding on a regular diet

In contrast to the long-term goals, short-term goals should address the immediate needs of the patient and should be accomplished within a short period of time (e.g., 2 to 4 weeks). Short-term goals might include

- prefeeding exercises

Exhibit 3-1 Functional Severity Levels for Dysphagia

Severe (nonfunctional)

- all nourishment by alternate feeding method
- NPO (i.e., prohibited from oral intake)
- trial oral intake, with physician's orders, by speech-language pathologist or feeding specialist only

Moderately severe (interferes with function)

- alternate feeding method still primary source of nourishment
- limited, inconsistent success with oral intake
- requires constant supervision
- some team involvement, but only speech-language pathologist or feeding specialist introduces new items or techniques

Moderate (interferes with function)

- alternate methods may be withdrawn on trial basis at this time
- fairly reliable with prescribed diet of specific items
- continues to require complete supervision
- nursing most involved, following instructions of speech-language pathologist or feeding specialist
- speech-language pathologist or feeding specialist working on addition of new items to patient's diet

Mild-moderate (interferes with function)

- fairly reliable with defined level of food consistency
- may still have difficulty with clear liquids or solids
- nursing staff takes primary responsibility for supervision of feeding
- self-feeding instruction initiated if upper extremity function permits

Mild (adequate but reduced)

- receives regular diet with only some foods restricted because of particular difficulty with them
- may still require some special techniques or procedures to achieve successful swallowing
- no longer requires close staff supervision

Minimal (adequate but reduced)

- receives a regular diet without any restrictions
- no supervision required
- occasional episodes of coughing with liquids or solids

Normal (adequate)

- independent in oral intake of all food consistencies
- safe and efficient swallowing competency

- direct swallowing therapy
- establishing compensatory techniques
- appropriate professional referrals for further evaluation and/or management

Procedures for the treatment of dysphagia are discussed in Chapter 6.

DISSEMINATING RESULTS OF THE DYSPHAGIA EVALUATION

The management of dysphagia requires a team approach that includes not only professionals such as the nurse, dietitian, and physician but also the patient and his or her family. Therefore, it is important that the feeding specialist be able to disseminate clearly and efficiently the results of the evaluation and recommended guidelines for feeding. Two alternate options are provided for this purpose. First, the CED has a face sheet on which suggestions for feeding, recommended diet, and precautions can be documented. This page can be duplicated and copies distributed to the appropriate team members. Second, a package of instructional handouts has been designed. The instructional handouts consist of three pages, which may be used individually or as a package:

- a simple diagram depicting normal swallowing
- a form for outlining the patient's specific problem areas
- a form listing the patient's recommended diet and individualized techniques to facilitate improved feeding

These handouts may be used to disseminate information in a variety of ways, including

- conveying evaluation results to appropriate team members
- outlining a treatment program to be carried out by nursing staff
- educating the patient and/or family about the normal swallowing process and conveying evaluation results to them
- providing patient or family members with an independent feeding program

Appendix 3-B includes some examples of completed instructional handouts.

SUMMARY

The CED is an essential first step in the overall management of dysphagia. Decisions to keep a patient NPO or to initiate oral feeding, recommendations for further evaluation of the swallow, or referrals to other medical professionals may all be based on the results of the clinical evaluation. Therefore, a comprehensive evaluation is essential. This chapter has discussed some guidelines for performing a clinical evaluation. The feeding specialist should adapt these guidelines to fit the needs and circumstances of the individual patient.

REFERENCES

Arms, R., Denes, D., & Tintsman, T. (1974). Aspiration pneumonia. *Chest, 65,* 136–139.

Bonanno, P. (1971). Swallowing dysfunction after tracheostomy. *Annals of Surgery, 174* (1), 29–33.

Cameron, J.L., Reynolds, J., & Zuidema, G.D. (1973). Aspiration in patients with tracheostomies. *Surgery, Gynecology and Obstetrics, 136,* 68–70.

Fleming, S.M. (1992). Treatment of mechanical swallowing disorders. In M.E. Groher (Ed.), *Dysphagia: Diagnosis and management,* 2nd ed., pp. 237–253. Stoneham, MA: Butterworth-Heinemann.

Hendrix, T.R. (1993). Art and science of history taking in the patient with difficulty swallowing. *Dysphagia, 8,* 69–73.

Hutchins, B.F., & Giancarlo, J.L. (1991). Developing a comprehensive dysphagia program. *Seminars in Speech and Language, 12* (3), 209–227.

Johnson, C.A., & Johnson, C.K. (1976). *Analysis of swallowing function in severe brain injury.* Paper presented at the American Speech, Language, Hearing Association, Houston.

Leopold, N.A., & Kagel, M.C. (1983). Swallowing ingestion and dysphagia: A reappraisal. *Archives of Physical Medicine and Rehabilitation, 64,* 371–373.

Linden, P., & Siebens, A. (1983). Dysphagia: Predicting laryngeal penetration. *Archives of Physical Medicine and Rehabilitation, 64,* 281–284.

Logemann, J. (1983). *Evaluation and treatment of swallowing disorders.* San Diego: College-Hill Press.

Miller, R.M. (1984). Evaluation of swallowing disorders. In M.E. Groher (Ed.), *Dysphagia: Diagnosis and management.* Stoneham, MA: Butterworth.

Miller, R.M. (1992). Clinical examination for dysphagia. In M.E. Groher (Ed.), *Dysphagia: Diagnosis and management* (2nd ed.). Stoneham, MA: Butterworth-Heinemann.

Muz, J., Mathog, R.H., Nelson, R., & Jones, L.A. (1989). Aspiration in patients with head and neck cancer and tracheostomy. *American Journal of Otolaryngology, 10,* 282–286.

Perlman, A., Langmore, S., Milanti, F., Miller, R., Mills, R.H., & Zenner, P. (1991). Comprehensive clinical examination of oropharyngeal swallowing function: Veterans Administration procedure. *Seminars in Speech and Language, 12* (3), 246–254.

Sasaki, C.T. (1980). Paralysis of the larynx and pharynx. *Surgical Clinics of North America, 60,* 1079–1092.

Sasaki, C.T., Suzuki, M., Horiuchi, M., & Kurchner, J.A. (1977). The effect of tracheostomy on the laryngeal closure reflex. *Laryngoscope, 87* (9), 1428–1433.

Steefel, J.S. (1981). *Dysphagia rehabilitation for neurologically impaired adults*. Springfield, IL: Charles C Thomas.

Stoschus, B., & Allescher, M.D. (1993). Drug-induced dysphagia. *Dysphagia, 8,* 154–159.

Weaver, A.W., & Fleming, S.M. (1978). Partial laryngectomy: Analysis of associated swallowing disorders. *American Journal of Surgery, 136,* 486–489.

APPENDIX 3-A

RIC Clinical Evaluation of Dysphagia (CED)

Leora Reiff Cherney, Ph.D., CCC-SP
Carol Addy Cantieri, M.A., CCC-SP
Jean Jones Pannell, MA., CCC-SP

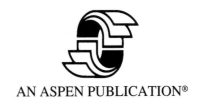

AN ASPEN PUBLICATION®

Clinical Evaluation of Dysphagia
Face Sheet

Patient: _____ Date: _____

Case #: _____ Clinician: _____

Overall diagnosis: _____
_____

Dysphagia severity: _____
_____

Suggestions for feeding: _____
_____
_____
_____
_____
_____
_____
_____
_____

Recommended diet: _____
_____
_____

Precautions: _____
_____
_____
_____
_____
_____
_____
_____
_____
_____
_____

Rehabilitation Institute of Chicago CED

Name: _____

Case #: _____

Date: _____

Evaluation of Prefeeding Skills

Medical/Nutritional Status _____

_____

_____

Respiratory Status _____

History of Aspiration _____

Tracheostomy _____ yes _____ no   Type _____   Size _____

    Position of Cuff _____ Inflated _____ Partially Inflated _____ Deflated

    Suctioning Required _____ yes _____ no   Frequency _____

    Other Relevant Information_____

Level of Responsiveness _____

Behavioral Characteristics _____

Current Feeding Method   Oral _____   Alternate _____

    Intake Amount _____   Frequency of Intake _____

    Other _____

Positioning

Habitual _____

Interfering Patterns _____

Trial/Optimal Position _____

_____

Observations of Oral, Pharyngeal, and Laryngeal Function

Lips _____

Tongue _____

Mandible _____

Rehabilitation Institute of Chicago CED

Dentition _____

Phonation _____

Articulation _____

Hypernasality _____   Hyponasality _____

Cough (involuntary and volitional) _____

Gag Reflex _____

Voluntary Swallow _____

Other Observations _____

Response to Stimulation

_____
_____
_____
_____
_____

Recommendations

_____ Swallowing Evaluation Deferred: Patient NPO

_____ Clinical Evaluation of Swallowing

_____ Videofluoroscopy

_____ ENT

_____ Other _____

_____

Goals:

_____
_____
_____
_____
_____
_____
_____
_____

Patient/Family Counseling:

_____
_____
_____

Name: _____

Case #: _____

Date: _____

General Impressions: _____

_____

Table columns (vertical headers): THIN LIQUIDS | THICK LIQUIDS | PUREED | GROUND SOLIDS | CHOPPED SOLIDS | REGULAR SOLIDS

I. *ORAL STAGE*

   A. *Lips*

   1. Protrusion

	Spoon	Cup	Straw
Initiates protrusion			
Maintains protrusion			

   _____ Initiates protrusion

   _____ Maintains protrusion

   2. Closure

   _____ Initiates Closure for Retrieval from Utensil

   _____ Maintains Closure for Retrieval from Utensil

   _____ Maintains Closure throughout Oral Stage

   _____ Leakage _____

   3. Interpretation of Lip Function

   _____ Adequate

   _____ Adequate but Reduced

   _____ Interferes with Function

   _____ Nonfunctional

   Problems due to

   _____ ↓ ↑ Tone

   _____ ↓   Sensation

   _____ ↓   Strength

   _____ ↓   Range of Motion

   _____ ↓   Rate

   _____   Inaccurate Direction

   _____   Other _____

   B. *Tongue*

   1. Bolus Formation and Transport

   _____ Adequate

   _____ Adequate but Reduced

   _____ Interferes with Function

   _____ Nonfunctional

   _____ Pumping Action of Tongue

   _____ Tongue Thrust

   2. Food Remaining in Mouth

   _____ None

   _____ Left Side

   _____ Right Side

   _____ Anterior

   _____ Roof of Mouth

   _____ Midline of Tongue

   _____ On Lips

Name: _____

Date: _____

THIN LIQUIDS
THICK LIQUIDS
PUREED
GROUND SOLIDS
CHOPPED SOLIDS
REGULAR SOLIDS

B. *Tongue* (cont.)
   3. Cough Reflex before Swallow
      _____ Yes
      _____ No
   4. Interpretation of Tongue Function
      _____ Adequate
      _____ Adequate but Reduced Function
      _____ Interferes with Function
      _____ Nonfunctional
      Problems due to
         _____ ↓ ↑ Tone
         _____ ↓ Elevation
         _____ ↓ Range of Motion Within Oral Cavity
         _____ ↓ External Range of Motion
         _____ ↓ Rate
         _____ ↓ Sensation
         _____ ↓ Strength
         _____ Inaccurate Direction
         _____ Other

C. *Mandible/Muscles of Mastication*
   1. Chewing
      _____ Rotary
      _____ Vertical
      _____ Absent
   2. Interpretation of Mandibular Function
      _____ Adequate
      _____ Adequate but Reduced Function
      _____ Interferes with Function
      _____ Nonfunctional
      Problems due to
         _____ ↓ ↑ Tone
         _____ Abnormal Reflexes (list)
         _____
         _____ ↓ Strength
         _____ ↓ Range of Motion
         _____ ↓ Rate
         _____ Dentition _____
         _____ Occlusion
         _____ Other

Rehabilitation Institute of Chicago CED

Name: _____

Date: _____

	THIN LIQUIDS	THICK LIQUIDS	PUREED	GROUND SOLIDS	CHOPPED SOLIDS	REGULAR SOLIDS

D. *Summary*

Overall Oral Phase

_____ Adequate

_____ Adequate but Reduced Function

_____ Interferes with Function

_____ Nonfunctional

Problems due to _____

_____

_____

Additional Comments: (Medical or behavioral status that *compensates* or *interferes* with performance)

_____

_____

_____

II. *PHARYNGEAL PHASE*

Gag Reflex   present   diminished   absent

Volitional Cough   present   diminished   absent

_____ Cough Reflex before Swallow

_____ Nasal Regurgitation

_____ Elevation of Hyoid and Thyroid Cartilage Observed

_____ Delayed Pharyngeal Swallow _____ seconds

_____ Repeated Swallows   Average number per bolus _____

_____ Complaints of Discomfort/Obstruction in Throat during

Swallow (specify location) _____

_____ Cough Reflex during Swallow

_____ Cough Reflex after Swallow

_____ Vocal Quality after Swallow

Describe _____

_____ Excessive Copious Secretions

_____ No Problems Exhibited

Rehabilitation Institute of Chicago CED

THIN LIQUIDS | THICK LIQUIDS | PUREED | GROUND SOLIDS | CHOPPED SOLIDS | REGULAR SOLIDS

Name: _____

Date: _____

A. *Summary*
    Overall Pharyngeal Phase
    _____ Adequate
    _____ Adequate but Reduced Function
    _____ Interferes with Function
    _____ Nonfunctional
    Problems due to_____
    _____
    _____
    _____

    Patient Appears Able/Unable to Protect Airway
    Additional Comments (e.g., medical or behavioral status that *compensates*
    or *interferes* with performance)_____
    _____
    _____
    _____

III. *ADDITIONAL TEST RESULTS*
      Videofluoroscopy Test Results/Recommendations

      _____
      _____
      _____
      _____
      _____
      _____
      _____

      ENT Test Results _____
      _____
      _____

      Other _____

IV. *OVERALL FUNCTIONAL SEVERITY LEVEL AND INTERPRETATION OF UNDERYLING
     NEUROMUSCULAR CHARACTERISTICS*

     _____
     _____
     _____
     _____
     _____

APPENDIX 3-B

Examples of Completed Instructional Handouts

Patient 1

This 43-year-old woman suffered a brain stem infarct with resultant left hemiparesis, left hemianesthesia, and left-sided 7th, 9th, 10th, and 12th cranial nerve paresis. The patient was being fed through a gastrostomy tube. She had a history (post-stroke) of recurrent aspirations.

In view of the patient's intact language skills, the instructional handout was given to her to supplement verbal explanations of her specific swallowing deficits and to outline specific swallowing techniques for secretion management. The Dysphagia Face Sheet was used to disseminate evaluation results and recommendations to the nursing floor.

Dysphagia Face Sheet

Patient: ___D.J._____   Date: ___5/93_____

Case #: ___1_____   Therapist: ___J.P._____

Overall diagnosis: ___Minimal flaccid dysarthria. Moderately severe dysphonia.___

Dysphagia severity: ___Severe dysphagia___

Suggestions for feeding: ___N.P.O.   Prefeeding program to be initiated by speech pathologists only___

Recommended diet: ___Continue G-tube feedings.___

Precautions: ___NPO___

Patient 1   *Name:* _____D.J._____

Schematic Drawing of Structures and Areas
Involved in the Swallowing Process

Soft Palate

Pharynx

Tongue

Epiglottis

Upper esophageal sphincter

Larynx

Esophagus

Vocal cords

Trachea

KATZ

To Stomach

To Lungs

Patient 1

Normal Feeding Process: *Name:* _____ D.J. _____
1. Food taken into mouth
2. Food chewed
3. Food moved to back of mouth
4. Swallow is initiated as follows:

   a) soft palate rises to block the nasal passageway
   b) muscles in the pharynx move the food downward (process of peristalsis)
   c) vocal cords in the larynx close to protect the airway
   d) upper esophageal sphincter opens, allowing food to pass into the esophagus
   e) upper esophageal sphincter closes to prevent regurgitation of food back into the pharynx and possibly the airway
   f) food continues through digestive tract by action of peristalsis

Malfunction of one or more of any of the following structures/processes can cause feeding difficulties.

Problem areas are circled and explained below:

LIPS   SOFT PALATE

TEETH   (PHARYNX)

MUSCLES OF CHEEK AND/OR   (VOCAL CORDS/OTHER
  JAW (FOR CHEWING)   LARYNGEAL MUSCLES

TONGUE   (UPPER ESOPHAGEAL SPHINCTER)

(INITIATION OF SWALLOW)   ESOPHAGUS

Description of Problems:

Swallow Initiation: The initiation of the swallow is delayed,
     resulting in delay of above steps 4a–f.
Pharynx: The action in step 4b is weakened and slower.
Vocal cords: The vocal cords are paralyzed in an open position, precluding the
     protective action of step 4c.
Upper esophageal sphincter: This sphincter is unable to open adequately
     precluding step 4d, and resulting in food piling up on top of the
     esophagus until it spills over through the vocal cords and into
     the lungs after the swallow.

Patient 1

Suggestions for Feeding: *Name:* _____ D.J. _____

1. Not ready to be fed. ___✓_____

2. Ready to be fed by the speech-language pathologist only. _____

3. Ready to be fed by nursing staff or family members familiar with the specific feeding program.
_____

4. Ready to self-feed with close supervision by trained staff and/or trained family members.
_____

5. Ready to self-feed with occasional supervision. _____

6. Independent self-feeding. _____

Recommended Diet:

Food consistencies to be used: _____ N.P.O. _____
_____

Food consistencies to be avoided: _____
_____

Feeding Techniques to Use:

Positioning: ___It will be easier for you to swallow sitting upright with your chin
_____tucked forward._____
_____

Presentation/placement of food: _____
_____N/A_____
_____

Other: _Use supraglottic swallow when swallowing your saliva: 1–Take breath._
2–Hold breath. 3–Swallow (hard). 4–Immediately cough (before you exhale or
inhale). 5–Swallow and breathe. **Practice laryngeal exercises as demon-
_strated during treatment sessions and outlined in your notebook._____

If you have any further questions, please contact: _____

Patient 2

This 20-year-old woman suffered an intracerebral hemorrhage caused by a blow to the head. A tracheostomy was performed in the acute care setting. At the time of the evaluation, the patient was alert, followed everyday conversation, and was being fed through a nasogastric tube.

She was found to exhibit a moderately severe dysphagia caused by cricopharyngeal dysfunction. Because she demonstrated limited success on thin liquids, a trial oral feeding program by the speech and language pathologist only was initiated. Within 3 weeks, the patient was ready for this program to be carried out by the nursing staff. The techniques were then demonstrated and the instructional handouts were used to explain further the nature of the dysphagia and specific feeding techniques to the nursing staff.

Name: _____K.B._____

Schematic Drawing of Structures and Areas
Involved in the Swallowing Process

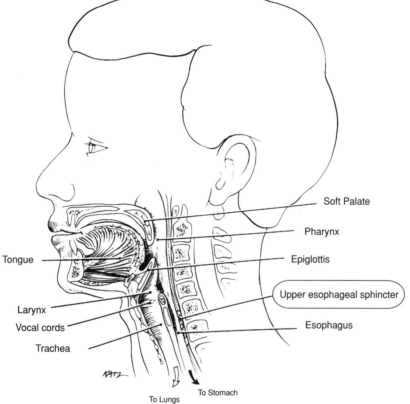

Patient 2

Normal Feeding Process: Name: _____K.B._____
1. Food taken into mouth
2. Food chewed
3. Food moved to back of mouth
4. Swallow is initiated as follows:

    a) soft palate rises to block the nasal passageway
    b) muscles in the pharynx move the food downward (process of peristalsis)
    c) vocal cords in the larynx close to protect the airway
    d) upper esophageal sphincter opens, allowing food to pass into the esophagus
    e) upper esophageal sphincter closes to prevent regurgitation of food back into the pharynx and possibly the airway
    f) food continues through digestive tract by action of peristalsis

Malfunction of one or more of any of the following structures/processes can cause feeding difficulties.

Problem areas are circled and explained below:

LIPS	SOFT PALATE
TEETH	PHARYNX
MUSCLES OF CHEEK AND/OR JAW (FOR CHEWING)	VOCAL CORDS/OTHER LARYNGEAL MUSCLES
TONGUE	(UPPER ESOPHAGEAL SPHINCTER)
INITIATION OF SWALLOW	ESOPHAGUS

Description of Problems:

    Upper esophageal sphincter does not open enough to allow food to pass into esophagus, but patient is able to swallow very small amounts (1/4 teaspoon) of thin liquids safely.

Patient 2

Suggestions for Feeding: *Name:* _____K.B._____

1. Not ready to be fed. _____

2. Ready to be fed by the speech-language pathologist only. _____

③ Ready to be fed by (nursing staff) or family members familiar with the specific feeding program.
_____✓_____

4. Ready to self-feed with close supervision by trained staff and/or trained family members.
_____

5. Ready to self-feed with occasional supervision. _____

6. Independent self-feeding. _____

Recommended Diet:

Food consistencies to be used: ___Thin liquids (¼ teasp. at a time)._____
_____

Food consistencies to be avoided: ___Nectars, purees, solids_____
_____

Feeding Techniques to Use:

Positioning: _____90° in chair_____
_____
_____

Presentation/placement of food: ¼ tsp. at a time via spoon. Wait 30 seconds after
patient swallows before presenting next spoonful. DO NOT give more than ¼
cup total.

Other: _Cuff should be deflated. Patient should temporarily occlude trach with
her finger during the swallow. Try to feed 3x/day for 15 minutes.
If excessive secretions and coughing noted, stop feeding and suction.
_____

If you have any further questions, please contact: _____

Patient 3

This 75-year-old man suffered a right hemisphere stroke with result-ant left hemiplegia, visual perceptual deficits, and left field neglect.

He also demonstrated a mild-moderate dysphagia. However, reduc-tions in function were primarily caused by cognitive and behavioral deficits, which significantly compounded oral motor functioning. Be-cause this patient required a consistent approach during mealtime, both the face sheet and instructional handouts were used to explain the dysphagia and its management to nursing staff, aides, and family.

Dysphagia Face Sheet

Patient: ___M.P.___ Date: ___1/12/93___

Case #: ___3___ Therapist: ___J.P.___

Overall diagnosis: ___Moderately severe communication deficit consistent with right hemisphere involvement.___

Dysphagia severity: ___Mild-moderate dysphagia___

Suggestions for feeding: ___Supervision___
    1—Low stimulus environment
    2—Serve one item at a time
    3—Small bites
    4—Verbally cue patient to swallow
    5—Verbally cue patient to put utensils down after each bite
    6—Verbally cue patient to clear left side of mouth

Recommended diet: ___Chopped solids and thick liquids___

Precautions: ___Patient's impulsive behavior requires supervision to ensure reduced rate of feeding and ingestion of small amounts, to prevent episodes of choking.___

Patient 3   *Name:* _____ M.P. _____

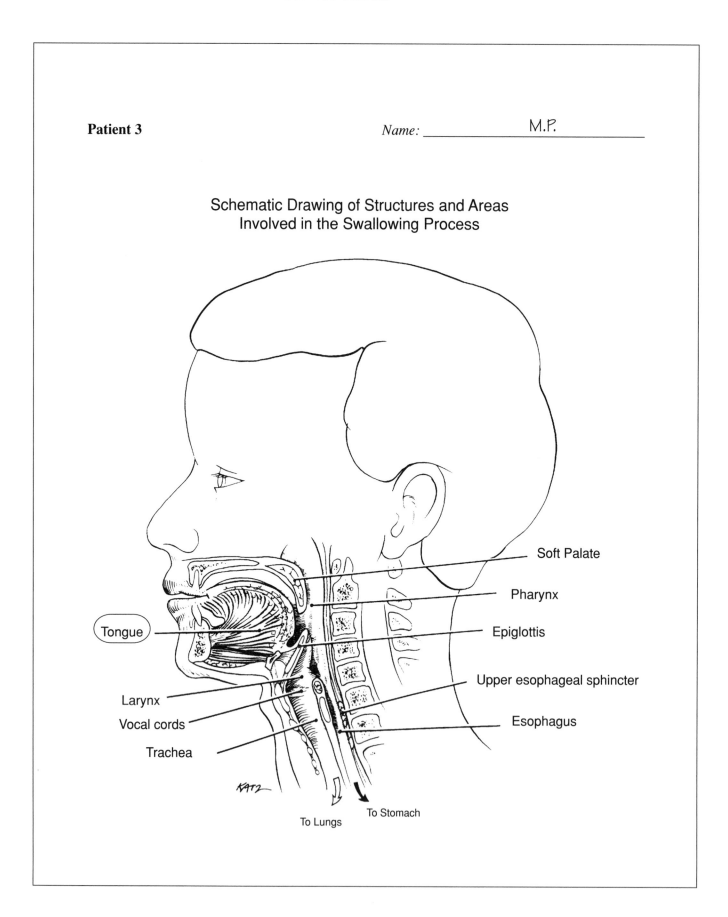

Schematic Drawing of Structures and Areas
Involved in the Swallowing Process

Patient 3

Normal Feeding Process: *Name:* _____M.P._____
1. Food taken into mouth
2. Food chewed
3. Food moved to back of mouth
4. Swallow is initiated as follows:

   a) soft palate rises to block the nasal passageway
   b) muscles in the pharynx move the food downward (process of peristalsis)
   c) vocal cords in the larynx close to protect the airway
   d) upper esophageal sphincter opens, allowing food to pass into the esophagus
   e) upper esophageal sphincter closes to prevent regurgitation of food back into the pharynx and possibly the airway
   f) food continues through digestive tract by action of peristalsis

Malfunction of one or more of any of the following structures/processes can cause feeding difficulties.

Problem areas are circled and explained below:

(LIPS)	SOFT PALATE
TEETH	PHARYNX
(MUSCLES OF CHEEK) AND/OR JAW (FOR CHEWING)	VOCAL CORDS/OTHER LARYNGEAL MUSCLES
(TONGUE)	UPPER ESOPHAGEAL SPHINCTER
(INITIATION OF SWALLOW)	ESOPHAGUS

Description of Problems:

Lips: Weakened, resulting in leakage.

Muscles of cheek: Weakened, resulting in pocketing of food on left side.

Tongue: Doesn't traffic food to the back of the mouth easily, resulting in food spilling out of the mouth, and food collecting in the mouth.

Swallow initiation: Slightly delayed, so that when patient takes food/ liquid in, he coughs.

*Behavior: impulsivity, reduced monitoring of amount of food put into mouth.

*Perceptual: Left field neglect, left side neglect.

Patient 3

Suggestions for Feeding: *Name:* _____M.P._____

1. Not ready to be fed. _____

2. Ready to be fed by the speech-language pathologist only. _____

3. Ready to be fed by nursing staff or family members familiar with the specific feeding program.
   _____

④ Ready to self-feed with close supervision by trained staff and/or trained family members.
   _____✓_____

5. Ready to self-feed with occasional supervision. _____

6. Independent self-feeding. _____

Recommended Diet:

Food consistencies to be used: ___Chopped solids and thick liquids_____
_____

Food consistencies to be avoided: ___Tough, stringy foods, thin liquids_____
_____

Feeding Techniques to Use:

Positioning: _____Upright at 90°_____
_____
_____

Presentation/placement of food: Small bites, one bite at a time (cue patient to set
utensil down after each bite); cue patient to swallow after each bite
_____

Other: Low stimulus environment_____
_____
_____
_____

If you have any further questions, please contact: _____

◆ CHAPTER 4 ◆

Clinical Assessment of Feeding and Swallowing in Infants and Children

Wendy S. Perlin and Maureen M. Boner

INTRODUCTION

The clinical evaluation of feeding and swallowing in infants and children includes the following:

- a preassessment in which the clinician gathers pertinent information regarding past and current factors affecting the feeding and swallowing process
- evaluation of sensory, motor, and structural components involved in the feeding and swallowing process. Sensation, symmetry, and tone of the face, lips, tongue, mandible, palate, and velopharynx are examined as well as dysmorphic features. Elicited movements of the oral musculature are also observed in either individual or repetitive movements
- observation of feeding and swallowing skills, while carefully controlling the amounts and consistencies of foods and liquids ingested
- recommendations for a videofluoroscopic (or other diagnostic imaging procedure) evaluation, if indicated

This chapter describes procedures for the

- preassessment
- sensory, motor, and structural evaluation
- observation of feeding and swallowing skills

Specific forms have been developed to guide the clinician through the clinical evaluation and to facilitate accurate documentation of the evaluation results. These forms are included in Appendix 4A. Chapter 5 provides further information about instrumental evaluation procedures such as videofluoroscopy and ultrasonography.

FEEDING PREASSESSMENT

Before presenting food or liquid, the clinician evaluates the child's readiness for oral feeding. This begins with a thorough history of the child's oral feeding skills, medical history, behavior, and other factors that affect the feeding and swallowing process. For example, some children who display oral motor skills that are within normal limits may not be cognitively or behaviorally ready to accept food or liquid. This may occur in children who are neurologically agitated or who have reduced levels of responsiveness. In other cases, individuals who have significant hypersensitivity or severe oral motor deficits may not be able to tolerate or physically manage food or liquid. An individual who has respiratory or cardiac involvement may have difficulty coordinating or maintaining breathing patterns during the feeding process.

The information gathered during the preassessment also helps the clinician determine the optimal situation in which to evaluate oral intake by the child (e.g., environment, positioning, food consistencies).

Parent/Caregiver Questionnaire

The *Parent/Caregiver Questionnaire* is designed to collect information for the preassessment. Regardless of whether the deficits are long-standing or recently acquired, the parent/caregiver can provide essential information about the following:

- history of feeding and swallowing problems
- typical feeding patterns and routines
- prior and present taste, temperature, and texture preferences
- parent/caregiver goals and/or concerns

Other important information can be obtained about

- typical positioning
- special utensils
- feeding techniques
- food preferences
- foods/liquids that are difficult for the child
- length of average feeding
- amount of food eaten per meal
- individuals who feel comfortable feeding the child

The questionnaire in Appendix 4A may be sent to the appropriate individual before the evaluation or it may be completed at the start of the evaluation in an interview format. The interview should be conducted in an informal, conversational manner to determine the *typical* feeding patterns. Questions may be paraphrased.

It is important to determine what the parent has been told previously about the child's feeding and swallowing problems. Also, it is *essential* to remain unbiased when the parent/caregiver is describing a feeding method that seems clinically inappropriate. These issues can be addressed later in the evaluation and during *subsequent* treatment and parent training sessions.

Preassessment Form

The *Preassessment Form* that the clinician fills out is based on information gathered from the parent/caregiver, teacher, therapists, physician, nurse, or medical chart. Check or comment on each of the following items that apply.

Behavior

It is important to note if the child's behavior is age-appropriate or if there are any behaviors that may potentially interfere with feeding. These behaviors may include

- reduced attention
- impulsivity
- fatigue
- agitation
- manipulative behaviors

Many behaviors interfere with overall tone, postures and positioning, which then make eating a more difficult and less efficient process.

- *Age-appropriate behavior*
  Determining age-appropriate behavior may be completed informally. Should the clinician desire a more formal measure of assessment, a variety of assessment tools are listed in Bailey and Woolery (1989) and Conner, Williamson, and Siepp (1978).
- *Reduced attention*
  A child with reduced attention may not be able to focus on the activity of eating. He or she may be easily distracted internally, by environmental stimuli, or by interaction with other people. Some children are distractible but may be easily redirected to the activity. Others may not be as easily refocused.
- *Impulsivity*
  An impulsive child may take too much food or liquid at one time. He or she may also take multiple bites of food or sips of liquid before swallowing. If a child puts too much food in his or her mouth, he or she may revert to less mature oral motor patterns to handle the large

amount. If a child is impulsive, present him or her with fewer food choices at a given time and provide greater structure to the situation.

- *Fatigue*
  The child may be fatigued prior to or at any point during the meal. The act of eating may be tiring in itself. Fatigue may cause the child to become irritable, to demonstrate less accurate and less mature oral skills, or to refuse to eat.
- *Agitation*
  Children may be in an agitated state of recovery after brain injury. Others may be agitated secondary to fatigue, frustration, or overstimulation. This can impede caregiver–child interaction, feeding patterns, attention to eating, or desire to eat.
- *Manipulation*
  Manipulative behaviors may also interfere with eating. These include refusal to eat, refusal to try new foods, refusal to participate, or refusal to follow directions. It is important to distinguish children who are behaviorally manipulative from those with sensory deficits. These two types of children often present with similar behaviors. Determining whether a child has sensory deficits is addressed during the sensorimotor evaluation.

Respiration

In the first year of life, breathing patterns progress from asynchrony between belly and upper chest breathing to abdominal breathing. Finally, mature thoracic breathing develops.

Evaluate the typical breathing pattern used (clavicular, thoracic, abdominal) and any changes seen in that pattern resulting from increased physical effort or fatigue. A variety of abnormal breathing patterns may be observed. These are described in Exhibit 4-1 and include

- periodic apnea
- gulp breathing
- gasp breathing
- reverse breathing
- asynchronous breathing
- stridorous breathing

Also, note whether general breathing is labored or has a raspy quality, or if the child is a habitual mouth-breather. Indicate whether there is a history of pulmonary or other medical problems interfering with respiration.

Tracheostomy Tubes

When evaluating a child who has a tracheostomy tube, determine the reason for the tracheostomy and the type, including fenestration, cuff, size, and brand. This can be done by checking the medical record and looking at the tracheostomy collar. Infants and small children will not have

Exhibit 4-1 Abnormal Breathing Patterns

Periodic apnea is characterized by shallow respiratory movements, with episodes of arrest. It is commonly seen in individuals with brain stem injury and central nervous system damage (McGee, 1987).

In **gulp breathing**, air is pushed into the lungs through the compression of the lips, cheeks, and tongue and the movement of the pharyngeal walls. This is seen in individuals who have extensive physical involvement or those in extreme distress (McGee, 1987).

Gasp breathing is characterized by an open-mouth posture and severe retraction of the tongue and head. This is seen when an already impaired system is overstressed (McGee, 1987).

Reverse breathing is a sign of severe respiratory distress and involves depression of the abdominal and thoracic areas simultaneously . Breathing can then only be accomplished through shoulder elevation. This pattern may be seen in individuals with asthma and with cystic fibrosis (McGee, 1987).

In **asynchronous breathing**, the thoracic cavity is depressed while the abdominal cavity expands, so that the sternum is drawn in at the area of the suprasternal notch. This pattern is often seen in individuals with low tone (McGee, 1987).

Stridorous breathing is characterized by audible inspirations and may be secondary to an ill-fitting tracheostomy tube, granulation tissue from prolonged intubation, vocal fold paralysis (unilateral or bilateral), or laryngeal webbing.

---

tracheostomy tubes with a cuff because of the relative size of the tracheostomy tube to the trachea. Ask the parent/caregiver, nurse, or physician how often suctioning is required or if the child has a productive cough that enables the child to clear secretions on his or her own. Determine if the child has a one-way valve or is able to be corked. Comment on the child's tolerance of these procedures. For more details regarding tracheostomy tubes, refer to Chapter 3.

Alternate Feeding

Children require nonoral feedings for a variety of reasons: swallowing problems, failure to thrive, reduced responsiveness, and other medical complications. Nasogastric (NG) tubes are generally used for a period of 3 to 6 months (Morris, 1989). However, NG tubes can be associated with reflux, sinusitis, increased gagging, and abnormal sensory input. Insertion of a tube through the nasopharynx prevents closure of the velopharynx, which decreases intraoral pressure. This ultimately interferes with sucking and swallowing (Morris, 1989). If the child requires nonoral feedings for an extended period of time, a gastrostomy tube or a jejunostomy tube will be placed (Moore & Green, 1985). However, gastrostomy tubes can also be associated with reflux (Wesley, Coran, Sarahan, Klein, & White, 1981). Determine the type of tube, the supplement given (formula type), amount per feeding, speed of feeding, and feeding schedule. It is particularly important to determine the recency of the feeding before the evaluation, as this may interfere with the child's state of hunger.

Positioning

Positioning directly affects the feeding process. A child's overall tone, gross motor, and fine motor abilities affect positioning during the feeding process. Observe and comment on the child's tone at rest and during volitional activities. Ask the parent/caregiver about the child's habitual feeding position and note which type of seating system is being used currently.

Once the child's habitual patterns have been evaluated, determine if changes from this position are necessary to assess optimal feeding conditions. Exhibit 4-2 describes further recommendations for position. It is advisable to work in coordination with an occupational or physical therapist to decide the optimal feeding position for the evaluation and subsequent treatment.

Interfering Patterns

Primitive reflexes and motor patterns may interfere with feeding. For example, the *asymmetric tonic neck reflex (ATNR)*, which is triggered by head turning to the side, results in flexion of the

---

Exhibit 4-2 Positioning Recommendations

Habitual Position for Feeding

The child's typical feeding position is usually the most efficient and successful for the parent/caregiver. This may not be the *optimal* position, but it is the position that the parent/caregiver is using. Modifying the feeding position is often a therapy goal. However, it is essential to observe the child being fed in the habitual position by the parent/caregiver. This enables the clinician to examine the child's habitual oral, motor, and swallowing skills.

Optimal Position for Feeding

In average children, feeding positions progress as the child's motor control (specifically head and trunk control) improves. Positions also change as the child's built-in protective mechanisms (normal physiologic development against aspiration) decrease. For the child with a recently acquired feeding disorder, always begin the evaluation in the optimal feeding position. From birth to 1 month of age, the infant is often supine with the head slightly elevated at an angle less than 45 degrees. At 3 months, the child is supported between 45 and 90 degrees. From 7 months on, the child is at 90 degrees, with varying amounts of support. A 7 month old needs moderate support, a 9 month old safety support only, and an 18 month old requires no support (Morris & Klein, 1987).

When a child presents with tonal abnormalities or specific oral-motor dysfunction, special care should be given to the feeding position as it may affect the child's performance in sucking, chewing, swallowing, and respiration. In general, the child should be well supported, with hips, knees, and ankles at 90 degrees to one another. When a child has particularly increased extensor tone, positioning him or her so that the hips are flexed greater than 90 degrees is helpful in breaking up the extensor pattern. The child's head should be at midline with a slight chin tuck. He or she should be in a relaxed state, with arms and hands near midline. Positioning should always be discussed and implemented with the input of a physical or occupational therapist, if available.

The feeder should sit directly in front of the child, a position that provides maximum interaction between the two and increased attention and focus on feeding. It is often helpful for the feeder to sit slightly below eye level of the child, so that the child will tend to look down, rather than up for presentation of the food. Looking down assists with appropriate chin-tuck posture. When working with an infant, it is appropriate to hold the child in such a way as to establish eye contact and achieve adequate tone control.

skull-side arm and extension of the face-side arm. Thus, the child may remain locked in this pattern, reducing his or her participation in the act of eating. Primitive reflex patterns are described in Chapter 2.

Children may exhibit compensatory patterns, such as hyperextension of the head, as part of an overall extension pattern or they may "fall" into hyperextension secondary to poor head control and ineffective positioning. Poor head control impedes the child's ability to keep the head in the optimal midline position. Overflow and compensatory patterns (including fixing and abnormal posturing) are more obvious during volitional movements, such as those required for eating.

Feeding Equipment

Determine the type of utensils and any adaptive equipment the child currently uses. If, during the evaluation, other utensils or adaptations are found to be more effective, make note of these.

Oral Intake

It is important to determine the typical foods and liquids a child ingests daily, as well as any difficulties or intolerances noted by the parent/caregiver.

- *Formula type*
  Determine whether the child is on formula, breast milk, or whole cow's milk. If the child is on formula, indicate the type and any additives (e.g., rice cereal).
- *Food type*
  If the infant is on food other than formula or milk, indicate the type (e.g., strained baby food).
- *Amount per feeding*
  Determine the amount of liquid and solid intake per average feeding.
- *Frequency of oral feeding*
  Indicate how often the child is fed (e.g., every 4 hours).
- *Duration*
  Estimate the length of an average feeding (e.g., 30 minutes).
- *History of intolerance*
  Indicate if the child has a history of food intolerance (e.g., allergies, lactose intolerance). Ask the parent/caregiver if the child has unusual episodes of emesis. For an infant, indicate if there is an unusual pattern of hiccups or burping at each meal, which may be indicative of reflux, acholasia, or incoordination between sucking and swallowing.

Medical Contraindicators

Determine if there are medical contraindicators such as

- fever
- history of aspiration
- respiratory, pulmonary, or cardiac complications

These can be obtained from the child's medical records or from the parent/caregiver and can be confirmed or clarified by the physician. If a child presents with a fever, determine the cause of the fever. Unexplained fevers are one symptom associated with aspiration pneumonia. Children with a history of gastroesophageal (G-E) reflux should be fed with careful attention to amounts of food given at one time, positioning during and after feeding, and increased risk of aspiration (Committee on Nutrition, American College of Pediatrics, 1985). Children with tracheoesophageal fistulas should not be fed. This opening between the walls of the trachea and the esophagus may result from treatment following head and neck cancer, traumatic injury to the tissue, or extensive intubation. Tracheomalacia is a softening of the tracheal tissues. It is usually a congenital condition that may interfere with the eating process secondary to respiratory problems. It may also follow prolonged intubation. Tracheal stenosis is a narrowing of the trachea and can result from a number of etiologies. Many times these children require tracheotomies for sufficient respiration.

Find out what types of medications the child is taking. Determine if these medications affect appetite, mental status, or behavior. Also determine if there are any diet restrictions because of allergies, diabetes, or other intolerances.

EVALUATION OF SENSATION, SYMMETRY, TONE, AND RELATED FEATURES

The evaluation of sensation, symmetry, tone, and elicited movements should be completed before presentation of food or liquid.

Sensation

Facial Sensation

If a child has reduced sensation, he or she may not be able to detect food residue or saliva on the face. If he or she is hypersensitive, the child may not let anyone touch the face, wash it, or remove food residue.

- Areas to assess
  1. Will the child allow touch to the face?
  2. Does he or she grimace or turn away when touched?
  3. Is the child unresponsive to touch?
  4. Can the child determine the site of touch (cheek versus chin)?
  5. Can he or she discriminate textures, such as rough, smooth, soft, or hard?

- Scoring procedure
  Indicate *N* for Normal, *R* for Reduced, or *E* for Excessive.

Labial Sensation

Reduced sensation in the lips may interfere with the child's ability to maintain closure while eating or drinking. It will impede the child's ability to sense the loss of food, liquid, or saliva.

Increased sensation/hypersensitivity in the lips may impede the child's acceptance of food or a utensil. He or she may be extremely reluctant to have anything come in contact with the lips.

- Areas to assess
  1. Will the child allow touch to the lips?
  2. Does he or she turn away, grimace or display no response when the lips are touched?
  3. Does the child attempt to wipe the lips when drool or food is present?
  4. If lips are touched, can he or she determine the site of touch?
  5. Does touching the lips trigger abnormal reflexes, such as ATNR or a startle?
  6. Does touching the lips trigger lip retraction, bite, or pucker?

- Scoring procedure
  Indicate *N* for Normal, *R* for Reduced, *E* for Excessive.

Lingual Sensation

A child who has increased sensation or hypersensitivity may not allow a utensil or food to be put into his or her mouth. If hypersensitive, a young child may reject a pacifier. A bite reflex may be triggered or tongue retraction may occur. Some children may exhibit a hyperactive gag when the anterior third of the tongue is touched.

- Areas to assess
  1. Is there a hyperactive gag?
  2. Is a bite reflex elicited?
  3. Is there tongue retraction?
  4. Does the child turn away or grimace when the tongue is touched?

- Scoring procedure
  Indicate *N* for Normal, *R* for Reduced, *E* for Excessive.

Palatal Sensation

Palatal sensation does not need to be addressed formally. A child with reduced sensation may be unaware of food packed in the palate. Hypersensitivity is not usually an isolated problem, and the child will probably resist any type food or liquid in the oral cavity.

- Scoring procedure
  Write any comments in the appropriate space on the evaluation form.

Velopharyngeal Sensation

A gag reflex is a normal reflex that occurs when the back of the pharynx is stimulated. Up to 40 percent of normal individuals do not have a gag reflex (Logemann, 1990). Children with neurologic problems may exhibit a hyperactive or hypoactive gag reflex.

- Area to assess
  Does the child exhibit a gag reflex after stimulation to the back of the pharynx?

- Scoring procedure
Check the appropriate description on the evaluation form.

Symmetry and Tone

Face

Symmetry: Symmetry is an important indicator of facial tone, active muscle control, and structural abnormalities.

- Areas to assess
Are the features symmetric?

- Scoring procedure
Indicate *N* for Normal/Symmetric or *D* for Deviant/Asymmetric. If the face is not symmetric, indicate the reason (e.g., surgical intervention, craniofacial anomalies, structural deviations) under the Comments sections.

Tone: Deviations in facial tone may not necessarily interfere with feeding and swallowing. However, decreased, increased, or fluctuating tone may be indicative of other neurologic problems (e.g., cranial nerve dysfunction).

- Areas to assess
1. At rest, does the child have normal, low, high, or fluctuating tone?
2. Does voluntary activity increase or change tone?

- Scoring procedure
Indicate *N* for Normal, *R* for Reduced, or *E* for Excessive. If tone fluctuates, print *Fluctuates*.

Related features

- Areas to assess
1. *Dysmorphic Features*: There are numerous types of dysmorphic features, many of which are associated with syndromes. Some examples of dysmorphic features include
   - epicanthic folds
   - hypertelorism (widely spaced eyes)
   - low set and rotated ears
   - ear pits
   - ear tags
   - unusual hair distribution
   - cleft (Sparks, 1984)

The presence of dysmorphic features alone may not directly interfere with eating but may be indicative of a syndrome with characteristics that do interfere with eating.

- Scoring procedure
List any observable dysmorphic features.

Lips

Symmetry: The child should have grossly symmetrical lips. If the lips are asymmetric, it may be due to changes in tone, muscle weakness, or structural deviations.

- Area to assess
  Are the lips symmetric?

- Scoring procedure
  Indicate *N* for Normal/Symmetric or *D* for Deviant/Asymmetric. If the lips are not symmetric, indicate the reason (e.g., surgical intervention, craniofacial anomalies, structural deviations, or muscle weakness).

Tone: Increased facial tone may cause grimacing, pursed lips, or a shortened upper lip. Decreased tone may lead to poor lip closure while eating. This will result in the loss of fluid or food.

- Area to assess
  Does the child have increased, decreased, or fluctuating tone in the lips?

- Scoring procedure
  Indicate *N* for Normal, *R* for Reduced, or *E* for Excessive. If tone fluctuates, print *Fluctuates*.

Related Features

- Areas to assess
  1. *Tremor:* Tremors are associated with breakdown in the consistent neural control of muscles (Darley, Aronson, & Brown, 1975). They can be seen at rest, but are sometimes present during movement, interfering with normal function.
  2. *Retraction:* Retraction of the lips may be secondary to hypersensitivity, an overflow of movement, or a compensatory or stabilizing/fixing pattern. Its presence will interfere with normal movement patterns.
  3. *Dysmorphic Features:* Possible features may include lip pits, indistinct filtrum, or a prominent cupid's bow. If other features are noted, list them.

- Scoring procedure
  Circle the items that apply and list any dysmorphic features seen.

Tongue

Symmetry: The tongue should be symmetric. Changes in symmetry may be due to tone, muscle weakness, or structural deviations.

- Area to assess
  Is the tongue symmetric?

- Scoring procedure
  Indicate *N* for Normal/Symmetric or *D* for Deviant/Asymmetric. If not symmetric, indicate the reason (e.g., surgical intervention, craniofacial anomalies, structural deviations, or muscle weakness).

Tone: While eating, reduced or increased tone in the tongue may impede manipulation of the bolus. Children who have cerebral palsy may present with a retracted tongue. Children with traumatic brain injury may present with increased tone in the tongue, which may cause tongue bunching. Reduced tone in the tongue may result in an undefined tongue shape, which makes the tongue appear larger in size and fill the oral cavity more completely.

- Area to assess
  Is there increased, decreased, or fluctuating tone?
- Scoring procedure
  Indicate *N* for Normal, *R* for Reduced, or *E* for Excessive. If tone fluctuates, print *Fluctuates.*

Related Features

- Areas to assess
  1. Look at the resting position of the tongue. Is it retracted, bunched, held in forward carriage, or does it deviate to one side?
  2. Is there atrophy, tremor, or fasciculation?
  3. Are there any dysmorphic features?
  4. Evaluate if the frenulum is too short and restricting tongue movement.

- Scoring procedure
  Circle items that apply and list any dysmorphic features seen.

Dentition/Mandible

Symmetry: The jaw should be symmetric.

- Area to assess
  Look closely at the child's bite. Does he or she have an overbite, underbite, or a crossbite?
- Scoring procedure
  Indicate whether the structure is *N* for Normal/Symmetric or *D* for Deviant/Asymmetric.

Related Features

- Areas to assess
  1. Does the individual have good oral hygiene?
  2. Are there excessive caries?
  3. Is there discoloration of the gums?
  4. Is a prosthesis in place?
  5. Are there missing or extra teeth (deciduous and/or adult)?
  6. Is there swelling of the gums?
  7. Does the child exhibit bruxism?

- Scoring procedure
  Circle or list any abnormalities. List any additional comments.

Palate

Determine if the individual has a cleft palate, submucosal cleft, repaired cleft, or a highly arched palate.

- Areas to assess
  1. Does the child have a high, flat, or normal arch?
  2. Does the child have a visible, repaired, or submucosal cleft?
- Scoring procedure
  Circle or list any abnormalities seen.

Velopharynx

Symmetry: Symmetry will be directly affected by tone. Asymmetry may also result secondary to post-tonsillectomy scarring (Darley et al., 1975). It may be difficult to view the velum in children who are very young or who are hypersensitive. Tongue positioning and tone may also interfere with assessment.

- Area to assess
  Is the velum symmetric at rest?
- Scoring procedure
  Indicate *N* for Normal/Symmetric and *D* for Deviant/Asymmetric. List the reason for asymmetry (tone or structural deviation).

Tone: Unilateral or bilateral tone deviations will affect symmetry and position of the velum. With unilateral weakness, the affected side rests at a lower level than the normal side. Bilateral weakness will result in both sides resting lower to the tongue base. In this case, a normally triggered gag will result in reduced or absent velopharyngeal movement (Darley et al., 1975). Children with increased tone or spasticity will present with narrowing of the velopharynx (Darley et al., 1975).

- Areas to assess
  Is velar tone within normal limits?
- Scoring procedure
  Indicate *N* for Normal, *R* for Reduced, *or E* for Excessive.

Related Features

- Areas to assess
  1. Is the uvula bifed? bifid
  2. Is there atrophy?
  3. Are the tonsils present or absent?
- Scoring procedure
  Comment on any abnormalities seen.

Pharynx and Larynx

Pharyngeal and laryngeal structures cannot be fully assessed during a clinical evaluation. When indicated, a full assessment should include a videoflouroscopic evaluation or other diagnostic imaging procedure.

Elicited Movements

The following areas can be assessed formally if the child will cooperate. Young children or more cognitively impaired children may not be able to complete this portion of the evaluation. Also, in the infant it is difficult to elicit specific performance of isolated movements. This is due to decreased comprehension of directions, difficulty with isolating motor movements, and difficulty performing on command. If the individual is unable to imitate or produce movements volitionally in a structured task, evaluate this area informally through play or observation. By evaluating elicited movements, one can determine whether there is apraxia, ataxia, weakness, reduced rate in repetitive movements, reduced organization of movements, or reduced ability to follow directions. Some children may require a model, such as a visual cue with a mirror, touch, or a verbal cue. However, if a child has significant difficulty with imitating or performing a movement and requires multiple cues, this may indicate poor motor planning, reduced initiation, or cognitive deficits.

Ask the child to complete each movement five or more times. If he or she is able to complete repetitive movements, circle *Repetitive*. If the child is only able to produce individual movements, circle *Individual* and evaluate performance on single movements. Decide whether the movements have adequate range, regular rate, adequate strength, and coordinated rhythm. Indicate in the Comments section what types of cues were provided for the child.

Lips

Retraction: Ask the child to smile. It should be a volitional smile rather than a reflexive smile.

- Areas to assess
  1. Is the range adequate bilaterally?
  2. Can the child smile at an efficient rate?
  3. Does the child demonstrate struggle patterns?
  4. Is there adequate strength to the movements?
  5. Are the movements coordinated?

- Scoring procedure
  Indicate *N* for Normal, *R* for Reduced, *E* for Excessive, and *I* for Irregular for left and right sides. Note any compensatory, abnormal, or overflow patterns observed in the Comments section.

Protraction: Ask the child to pucker the lips.

- Areas to assess
  1. Is the range adequate bilaterally?
  2. Can the individual pucker at an efficient rate?

3. Are there struggle patterns?

4. Is there adequate strength to the movements?

5. Are the movements coordinated?

- Scoring procedure

  Indicate *N* for Normal, *R* for Reduced, *E* for Excessive, and *I* for Irregular for left and right sides. Note any compensatory, abnormal, or overflow patterns observed in the Comments section.

Compression: Ask the child to put the lips together tightly and then release. To assess strength, ask the child to resist your attempt to pull the lips apart.

- Areas to assess

  1. Is the range adequate bilaterally?

  2. Can the individual compress the lips at an efficient rate?

  3. Are there struggle patterns?

  4. Is there adequate strength to the movements?

  5. Are the movements coordinated?

- Scoring procedure

  Indicate *N* for Normal, *R* for Reduced, *E* for Excessive, and *I* for Irregular for left and right sides. Note in the Comments section any compensatory, abnormal, or overflow patterns observed.

Tongue

Lateralization: Ask the child to lateralize the tongue from right to left outside of the mouth.

- Areas to assess

  1. Is the range adequate bilaterally?

  2. Can the child lateralize at an efficient rate?

  3. Are there struggle patterns?

  4. Is there adequate strength to the movements?

  5. Are the movements coordinated?

- Scoring procedure

  Indicate *N* for Normal, *R* for Reduced, *E* for Excessive, and *I* for Irregular, for left and right sides. Note in the Comments section any compensatory, abnormal, or overflow patterns observed.

Cheek Pushes: Ask the child to push with the tongue against the inside of each cheek.

- Areas to assess

  1. Is the range adequate bilaterally?

  2. Are there struggle patterns?

  3. Is there adequate strength to the movements?

  4. Are the movements coordinated?

- Scoring procedure
  Indicate *N* for Normal, *R* for Reduced, *E* for Excessive, and *I* for Irregular for left and right sides. Note any compensatory, abnormal, or overflow patterns observed in the Comments section.

Circular Range of Motion: Ask the child to move the tongue in a circular pattern around the lips, as if he or she were cleaning them.

- Areas to assess
  1. Is the range adequate bilaterally?
  2. Can the child circle the lips at an efficient rate?
  3. Are there struggle patterns?
  4. Is there adequate strength to the movements?
  5. Are the movements coordinated?

- Scoring procedure
  Indicate *N* for Normal, *R* for Reduced, *E* for Excessive, and *I* for Irregular for left and right sides. Note any compensatory, abnormal, or overflow patterns observed in the Comments section.

Protrusion: Ask the child to stick out the tongue.

- Areas to assess
  1. Is the range adequate?
  2. Can the child protrude the tongue at an efficient rate?
  3. Are there struggle patterns?
  4. Is there adequate strength to the movement?
  5. Are the movements coordinated?

- Scoring procedure
  Indicate *N* for Normal, *R* for Reduced, *E* for Excessive, and *I* for Irregular. Note in the Comments section any compensatory, abnormal, or overflow patterns observed.

Elevation Outside the Lips: Ask the child to protrude and then elevate the tongue. The child may need cues to lower the mandible and avoid using the lips to assist.

- Areas to assess
  1. Is the range adequate?
  2. Can the child elevate the tongue at an efficient rate?
  3. Are there struggle patterns?
  4. Is there adequate strength to the movement?
  5. Are the movements coordinated?

- Scoring procedure
  Indicate *N* for Normal, *R* for Reduced, *E* for Excessive, and *I* for Irregular. Note in the Comments section any compensatory, abnormal, or overflow patterns observed.

Elevation to Hard Palate: Ask the child to elevate the tongue to touch the roof of the mouth.

- Areas to assess
  1. Is the range adequate?
  2. Can the child elevate the tongue at an efficient rate?
  3. Are there struggle patterns?
  4. Is there adequate strength to the movement?
  5. Are the movements coordinated?

- Scoring procedure
  Indicate *N* for Normal, *R* for Reduced, *E* for Excessive, and *I* for Irregular. Note in the Comments section any compensatory, abnormal, or overflow patterns observed.

Depression: Ask the child to depress the tongue outside the lips.

- Areas to assess
  1. Is the range adequate?
  2. Can the child depress the tongue at an efficient rate?
  3. Are there struggle patterns?
  4. Is there adequate strength to the movement?
  5. Are the movements coordinated?

- Scoring procedure
  Indicate *N* for Normal, *R* for Reduced, *E* for Excessive, and *I* for Irregular. Note in the Comments section any compensatory, abnormal, or overflow patterns observed.

Dentition/Mandible

Ask the child to open and close the mouth. Carefully observe for actual mandibular movement versus abnormal compensatory labial and lingual movement.

- Areas to assess
  1. Is the range adequate?
  2. Can the child open and close the mouth at an efficient rate?
  3. Are there struggle patterns?
  4. Is there adequate strength to the movement?
  5. Are the movements coordinated?

- Scoring procedure
  Indicate *N* for Normal, *R* for Reduced, *E* for Excessive, and *I* for Irregular. Note in the Comments section any compensatory, abnormal, or overflow patterns observed.

Velopharynx

Velopharyngeal movement can be assessed during phonation. Ask the child to say "ah" repeatedly.

- Areas to assess
  1. Is the range adequate bilaterally?
  2. Can the child say "ah" at an efficient rate?
  3. Are there struggle patterns?
  4. Are the movements coordinated?
  5. Is there adequate strength to the movement?
  6. Is vocal quality hypernasal or hyponasal?

- Scoring procedure
  Indicate *N* for Normal, *R* for Reduced, *E* for Excessive, and *I* for Irregular, for left and right sides. Check vocal quality on the form. Note in the Comments section any compensatory, abnormal, or overflow patterns observed.

Pharynx/Larynx

Assess whether the child's own secretions appear to be pooling in the valleculae, pyriform sinuses, or resting on the vocal cords, before presenting any type of food or liquid. This can sometimes be determined by the presence of wet vocal quality during phonation. Also, assess whether the child displays adequate laryngeal elevation on a dry swallow. Laryngeal elevation is minimal in infants. It is more clearly detectable in children. Laryngeal elevation can be clinically assessed in a child by placing two fingers on the larynx and asking the child to swallow. A rapid upward and slightly forward movement should be felt. The movement does not ensure airway protection but indicates laryngeal movement. Airway protection can be determined by videofluoroscopy.

- Areas to assess
  1. Is there an abnormal wet vocal quality when the child's head is in midline?
  2. Is there wet vocal quality after the child tilts the head back? (Logemann, 1989).
  3. Can the child clear wet vocal quality, if noted?
  4. Is there wet vocal quality after the child rotates the head left and right? (Logemann, 1989).
  5. Does the child display adequate laryngeal elevation?

- Scoring procedure
  Indicate whether the vocal quality is clear or wet. Comment on the child's ability to clear secretions if they are present. Indicate *P* for Present, *A* for Absent, and *R* for Reduced laryngeal elevation.

EVALUATING ORAL INTAKE

When assessing infants and children, it is important to remember that their performance will depend on their age, level of cognition, behavior, and comfort level. The evaluation of infants and young children should be completed informally and playfully, during a meal when possible. Before and during the evaluation, explain to the child and parent/caregiver what you are doing and why. When evaluating the child with long-standing deficits, have the parent/caregiver feed the child for a portion of the evaluation. This will give the clinician a general idea of habitual feeding interactions, as well as comfort the child in a potentially unfamiliar setting.

Children with recently acquired deficits, who are being fed orally for the first time, should be fed by the clinician only. However, every effort should be made to include the parent/caregiver in the evaluation.

Environment

If possible, conduct the evaluation in both the child's habitual and optimal environments so that performance can be determined in each setting. The optimal environment is distraction-free. This enables the child to focus on the feeding process, thereby maximizing his or her performance. When attempting to recreate the habitual environment, consider the typical surroundings, food and liquid consistency and temperature, and parent/caregiver.

The child being fed for the first time should be fed in the optimal environment. If the child does well in the optimal environment, introduce distractions that are typical of the child's environment. Determine which distractions have the greatest impact on the feeding process.

Preparations

Have all food and utensils ready before the evaluation begins. If appropriate, ask the parent/caregiver to bring food and feeding equipment that the child likes and typically uses. Different types of food and utensils will be necessary for each child. For example, a child with a tracheostomy tube who is on trial feedings or has been fed non-orally (NPO) will not need a full variety of foods for the initial evaluation. The only consistencies needed may be pureed food and thin and thick liquids that have been dyed blue. An evaluation for another child may include thin and thick liquids, pureed food, ground food, soft chopped food, and regular food. An infant will require his or her formula and different types of baby food. During the assessment, give the child some choices in the foods he or she eats.

Tools we suggest you have on hand include

- latex or maroon spoons
- metal utensils
- tippy cup
- cut-out cup
- regular cup
- bowls
- plates
- straws
- a variety of infant and premie nipples
- NUK brushes

- bottles
- pen light
- towels and bibs

There is a complete resource guide of feeding utensils listed in Morris and Klein (1987). Gloves will also be needed to comply with use of body substance isolation (BSI) precautions. These precautions require the use of hand washing, eye protection, and gloves when there is the possibility of contact with any body substance. This includes saliva, mucus, blood, and other body substances.

When presenting food or liquid to a child, start by using a latex spoon or a NUK brush unless the parent/caregiver has had success with a more familiar utensil. Metal spoons may stimulate a bite reflex. There is also the danger that a child may bite down on a plastic spoon or tongue depressor, causing it to break off in his or her mouth. If there is no evidence of a bite reflex, you may switch to a plastic or metal spoon.

PEDIATRIC SCALE

The *Pediatric Scale* looks at performance related only to the acts of eating and drinking. As with other milestones, oral motor abilities follow a general developmental progression, with a broad range of normal. The normal developmental feeding milestones are discussed in Chapter 2. The purpose of this scale is to guide the clinician in determining whether the infant or child's feeding milestones are age appropriate.

Reflexes

Infants are born with a set of reflexes that are basic to survival. Most of these reflexes are assimilated as the infant develops more control over his or her body and the environment. Neurologically impaired children may continue to exhibit these reflexes beyond the normal developmental stage. The persistence of these reflexes limit the child's development in all areas, including feeding and swallowing. When scoring this section, "present" indicates that a pattern or skill is consistently observed. As a child develops, some less mature patterns begin to fade and are only apparent "some of the time." More mature patterns begin to "emerge" but are not seen consistently. Refer to Chapter 2 (Exhibit 2-1) to determine ages when these reflexes are appropriate.

Rooting

- Area to assess
  Elicit the rooting reflex by touching the child's cheek near the corner of the mouth. He or she should automatically turn toward your hand in search of nipple or bottle.

- Scoring procedure
  Indicate *P* for Present, *P** for Present some of the time, *EM* for Emerging, or *A* for Absent.

Babkin

- Area to assess
  Deep pressure to the palm of the hand results in the infant opening the mouth, closing the eyes, and bringing the head forward.

- Scoring procedure
  Indicate *P* for Present, *P** for Present some of the time, *EM* for Emerging, or *A* for Absent.

Palmomental

- Area to assess
  Similar to the Babkin, the palmomental reflex is elicited by touching the palm of the hand. This causes the chin to wrinkle.

- Scoring procedure
  Indicate *P* for Present, *P** for Present some of the time, *EM* for Emerging, or *A* for Absent.

Transverse Tongue

- Area to assess
  When stimulated laterally by touch or taste, the tongue moves in the direction of the stimulus.

- Scoring procedure
  Indicate *P* for Present, *P** for Present some of the time, *EM* for Emerging, or *A* for Absent.

Bite

- Area to assess
  This is a rhythmic series of up-and-down jaw movements produced after tactile stimulation to the teeth or gums.

- Scoring procedure
  Indicate *P* for Present, *P** for Present some of the time, *EM* for Emerging, or *A* for Absent.

Gag

- Area to assess
  Stimulation to the posterior half of the oral cavity results in mouth opening, head extension, and the floor of the mouth depressing.

- Scoring procedure
  Indicate *P* for Present, *P** for Present some of the time, *EM* for Emerging, or *A* for Absent.

Startle

- Area to assess
  This reflex is elicited by pushing a child backward while in supported sitting or by making a loud noise. The child reflexively extends and abducts the arms and legs.

- Scoring procedure

    Indicate *P* for Present, *P** for Present some of the time, *EM* for Emerging, or *A* for Absent.

Grasp

- Area to assess

    The grasp reflex is elicited as the adult places his or her finger across the infant's palm, giving a slight pull. The baby grasps and holds onto the finger.

- Scoring procedure

    Indicate *P* for Present, *P** for Present some of the time, *EM* for Emerging, or *A* for Absent.

Asymmetric Tonic Neck Reflex

- Areas to assess

    While the child is placed in supine, turn his or her head to the side and watch for extension of the arm on the child's face side and flexion of the arm on the skull side. This should be elicited on both sides.

- Scoring procedure

    Indicate *P* for Present, *P** for Present some of the time, *EM* for Emerging, or *A* for Absent.

Neck Righting Reaction

- Area to assess

    The neck righting reaction is elicited by turning the head to the side in supine. This results in the body following behind the head turn. The body moves as one unit, much like a log roll.

- Scoring procedure

    Indicate *P* for Present, *P** for Present some of the time, *EM* for Emerging, or *A* for Absent.

Face

Varied Facial Expressions

- Area to assess

    Observe what type of behaviors in the parent/caregiver (e.g., intonation, facial expression, volume) elicit changes in expression. Note the type and frequency of the infant's reaction.

- Scoring procedure

    Indicate *P* for Present, *P** for Present some of the time, *EM* for Emerging, or *A* for Absent.

Recognition of Utensil

Before feeding, present the bottle, cup, and/or spoon one at a time to the child.

- Area to assess

    Does the child change his or her expression or increase the activity level, demonstrating recognition of these items?

- Scoring procedure
  Indicate *P* for Present, *P** for Present some of the time, *EM* for Emerging, or *A* for Absent.

Anticipation

Watch the child's responses as you prepare for the feeding session (e.g., take the lid from the bottle to add chosen liquid, remove the top from a jar of baby food). Make sure the infant is able to see the preparation.

- Areas to assess
  1. Does his or her activity level increase?
  2. Does the child seemingly "reach" for you or the food or drink?
  3. Does the child appear eager and know that he or she is about to be fed?

- Scoring procedure
  Indicate *P* for Present, *P** for Present some of the time, *EM* for Emerging, or *A* for Absent.

Lips

In each stage of eating or drinking during the evaluation, watch lip movement.

- Areas to assess
  1. Are the lips approximated at rest?
  2. Do they approximate around the bottle, cup, spoon, fork, or finger foods?
  3. Do they actively close and maintain the position for increased sucking or food removal?
  4. Does the infant's suck increase and is there active pull on nipple to maintain the bottle when you attempt to remove it?
  5. Is lip closure maintained over time during the meal, or is it present initially and then decreased?
  6. Is there any food or liquid lost from the corners of the mouth because of poor lip closure?
  7. Is the child able to remove food from the utensil?

- Scoring procedure
  Indicate *P* for Present, *P** for Present some of the time, *EM* for Emerging, or *A* for Absent.

Tongue

The tongue serves multiple functions during the oral intake process (e.g., shaping the bolus, propelling food posteriorly for swallowing, lateralizing to keep food on the molars/gum ridge for chewing). Tongue movement follows a developmental progression and varies according to the textures of food presented.

- Areas to assess
  1. On opening the mouth in anticipation of food, is there a cupped configuration of the anterior and central portions of the tongue?

2. When the child swallows, does the tongue tip protrude beyond the teeth?

3. Is any lateralization of the tongue seen when textured foods are presented laterally?

4. Does the child exhibit lingual skills necessary to form a bolus?

5. Is the bolus moved posteriorly in a timely fashion before the swallow?

6. Does the child demonstrate the ability to clean remaining food/liquid from the lips using the tongue?

- Scoring procedure

Indicate *P* for Present, *P** for Present some of the time, *EM* for Emerging, or *A* for Absent.

Dentition/Mandible

As noted in Chapter 2, mandibular control progresses from significant excursion to controlled, regular movements and ability to determine strength needed for biting/chewing. When observing the child, note the excursion.

- Areas to assess

1. Do the tongue and jaw move separately or as one unit?

2. Are the movements rhythmic?

3. Is the child able to bite off a cookie or cracker in a single, graded movement?

4. Are external controls, such as the edge of a cup, used to achieve jaw stability?

5. Is a munching/vertical chew pattern (where food must be placed directly between the molars/gum ridge to be processed) used?

6. Is a rotary chewing pattern used?

7. Is chewing initiated and maintained?

- Scoring procedure

Indicate *P* for Present, *P** for Present some of the time, *EM* for Emerging, or *A* for Absent.

Coordination

Feeding skills require coordination between oral motor and respiratory systems.

- Areas to assess

1. Is the predominant pattern a suck or suckle when the infant is drinking from a bottle or breast or when the child drinks from the cup?

2. Is the pattern active or achieved through jaw excursion and positioning along with infant "fat pads" in the cheeks?

3. How many times is the infant able to suck/suckle before taking a breath?

4. Is a full pause needed to accomplish the breath?

- Scoring procedure

Indicate *P* for Present, *P** for Present some of the time, *EM* for Emerging, or *A* for Absent.

SUMMARY OF FEEDING AND SWALLOWING PATTERNS

The results of the evaluation are compiled on the *Summary of Feeding and Swallowing Patterns.* This form allows the clinician to document the functional feeding and swallowing performance for each of six food consistencies. Information from the *Preassessment* and oral examination are summarized briefly as they relate to the feeding process. Careful consideration of the developmental feeding and swallowing skills of the child (as documented on the *Pediatric Scale*) permits a more accurate interpretation of the results and appropriate delineation of treatment goals.

General Impressions

Comment on general impressions, interaction between the child and caregiver, interfering patterns and behaviors, and the child's response to the feeding process.

Lips

Delay in skill development or deviant skills displayed during completion of the *Pediatric Scale* may result in difficulty in the functional feeding process. For example, poor lip closure often results in loss of liquid or food.

- Scoring procedure
  If the child displays skills appropriate to his or her developmental level, check *No Problems Exhibited.* Any abnormal patterns observed should be checked in the appropriate column for the specific texture.

Tongue

Poor lingual function may result in liquid or food remaining in the oral cavity. This residue is often pooled in the anterior or lateral sulci, packed in the palate, or pocketed in the cheeks. Tongue thrusting or tongue extrusion may force food or liquid out of the oral cavity. Tongue retraction may interfere with placement of food or liquid and results in pooling of material in the oral cavity. Each of these abnormal patterns will interfere with oral transit time.

- Scoring procedure
  If the child displays skills appropriate to his or her developmental level, check *No Problems Exhibited.* Any abnormal patterns observed should be checked in the appropriate column for the specific texture. *The time for delayed oral transit should be noted.*

Dentition/Mandible

Abnormal patterns in mandibular movement interfere in a variety of ways. Jaw thrust or strong extension of the jaw interferes with adequate grading of jaw opening. This may interfere with placement of the liquid or food and result in loss of material from the oral cavity. Tonic bite reflex may be triggered by contact of a utensil with the face, lips, teeth, or tongue. The trigger site will vary with each child and may not be consistently present. Jaw clenching may result from the tonic bite reflex, from hypersensitivity, or as a learned behavior secondary to the need for multiple invasive medical procedures (Morris & Klein, 1987). These patterns may interfere with acceptance of the utensil in the oral cavity, accurate placement of liquid or food, or removal of the utensil. Munching or vertical chewing patterns result in poor mastication of food. Rather than using the mature diagonal/rotary movement of the jaw, simple up and down movements are seen. Reduced tongue lateralization further results in the child's inability to maintain the food on the surface of the teeth for chewing. Bruxism may or may not interfere with the feeding process. This pattern may interfere with acceptance of the utensil. At times, after masticating the food, the child will continue to grind the teeth nonfunctionally.

- Scoring procedure
  If the child displays skills appropriate to his or her developmental level, check *No Problems Exhibited*. Any abnormal patterns observed should be checked in the appropriate column for the specific texture.

Swallowing

During administration of the *Pediatric Scale*, different swallowing problems may have been observed. Reduced oral sensation or reduced range, strength, or coordination of lingual movement may result in material dripping over the back of the tongue into the pharynx, which pools in the valleculae. The child may also display a delayed or absent pharyngeal swallow, resulting in pooling of material in the valleculae. These patterns may result in wet vocal quality or coughing before the swallow. Reduced pharyngeal peristalsis may result in material resting in the valleculae and pyriform sinuses, possibly leading to aspiration after the swallow. The child may display a wet vocal quality or cough after the swallow has triggered. The child may compensate for reduced lingual movement or residue in the pharynx by producing multiple swallows per bolus. With reduced laryngeal closure, material may enter the airway, resulting in coughing during the swallow. Reduced laryngeal elevation may result in coughing or wet vocal quality after the swallow (Logemann, 1983). It should be noted that some children may silently aspirate without displaying wet vocal quality or a cough. To determine if there is material resting in the valleculae, have the child tilt the head back, emptying the material into the pharynx and listen for a wet vocal quality or cough. To determine if material is resting in the pyriform sinuses, have the child turn the head to the left and right, clearing the sinuses and listen for a wet vocal quality or cough (Logemann, 1989). To determine where specific breakdown in the swallowing process occurs, a videofluoroscopic or other diagnostic imaging procedure is necessary.

- Scoring procedure
  If the child displays skills appropriate to his or her developmental level, check *No Problems*

Exhibited. Any abnormal patterns observed should be checked in the appropriate column for the specific texture. The time for delayed trigger of the pharyngeal swallow should be listed. The number of swallows per bolus should also be recorded.

Results

Discuss the functional deficit areas and developmental age level, when appropriate.

Recommendations

Document any diagnostic recommendations (e.g., videofluoroscopy, ultrasonography) and prescribed intervention techniques. When devising the treatment plan, the following areas, which are discussed in Chapter 7, should be considered:

- environment for feeding
- position
- recommended feeders
- recommended utensils
- treatment techniques or strategies
- prescribed textures of liquids and foods
- prescribed amounts of liquids and foods

REFERENCES

Bailey, D., & Woolery, M. (1989). *Assessing infants and preschoolers with handicaps.* Columbus OH: Merrill.

Committee on Nutrition, American Academy of Pediatrics. (1985). *Pediatric nutrition handbook.* In G. Forbes & C. Woodruf (Eds). Elk Grove Village, IL: American Academy of Pediatrics.

Connor, F., Williamson, G., & Siepp, J. (Eds.). (1978). *Program guide for infants and toddlers with neuromotor and other developmental disabilities.* New York: Teachers' College Press.

Darley F., Aronson, A., & Brown, J. (1975). *Motor speech disorders.* Philadelphia: W. B. Saunders.

Logemann, J. (1983). *Evaluation and treatment of swallowing disorders.* San Diego, CA: College-Hill Press.

Logemann, J. (1989). Evaluation and treatment planning for the head-injured patient with oral intake disorders. *Journal of Head Trauma Rehabilitation, 4* (4), 24–33.

Logemann, J. (1990). *Infant swallowing.* Miniseminar presented at the meeting of the Illinois Speech-Language-Hearing Association, Chicago, Illinois.

McGee, M. (1987). *NeuroDevelopmental treatment: Pediatric certification course.* Winston-Salem, North Carolina

Moore, M. C., & Green, H. L. (1985). Tube feeding of infants and children. *Pediatric Clinics of North America, 32*(2), 401–417.

Morris, S. (1989). Development of oral-motor skills in the neurologically impaired child receiving non-oral feedings. *Dysphagia, 3,* 135–154.

Morris, S., & Klein, M. (1987). *Pre-feeding skills.* Tucson, AZ: Therapy Skill Builders.

Sparks, S. (1984). *Birth defects and speech-language disorders*. San Diego, CA: College-Hill Press.

Wesley, J., Coran, A., Sarahan, T., Klein, M., & White, S. (1981). The need for evaluation of gastroesophageal reflux in brain damaged children referred for feeding gastrostomy. *Journal of Pediatric Surgery, 16* (6), 866–870.

SUGGESTED READINGS

Bosma, J., Donner, M., & Tanaka, E. (1986). Anatomy of the pharynx. *Dysphagia, 1,* 23–33.

Bosma, J., Donner, M., Tanaka, E., & Robertson, D. (1986). Anatomy of the pharynx, pertinent to swallowing. *Dysphagia, 1,* 23–33.

Buchholz, D., Bosma, J., & Donner, M. (1985). Adaptation, compensation, and decompensation of the pharyngeal swallow. *Gastrointestinal Radiology, 10,* 235–239.

Casaer, P., Daniels, H., Devlieger, H., DeCock, P., & Eggermont, E. (1982). Feeding behavior in preterm neonates. *Early Human Development, 7,* 331–346.

Cherney, L., Cantieri, C., & Pannell, J. (1986). *Clinical evaluation of dysphagia*. Rockville, MD: Aspen Publishing Company.

Christensen, J. (1989). Developmental approach to pediatric neurogenic dysphagia. *Dysphagia, 3,* 131–134.

Cowett, R., Lipsitt, B., & Oh, W. (1978). Aberrations in sucking behavior of low-birthweight infants. *Developmental Medicine and Child Neurology, 20,* 701–709.

Daniels, H., Caeser, P., Devlieger, H., & Eggermont, E. (1986). Mechanisms of feeding efficiency in preterm infants. *Journal of Pediatric Gastroenterology and Nutrition, 5,* 593–596.

Darwin, C. (1971). A biographical sketch of an infant. *Mind, 24,* 3–8.

Di Scipio, W., Kaslon, K., & Ruben, R. (1978). Traumatically acquired conditioned dysphagia in children. *Annals of Otology, 87,* 509–514.

Dubignon, J. & Cooper, D. (1980). Good and poor feeding behavior in the neonatal period. *Infant Behavior and Development, 3,* 395–408.

Finnie, N. (1975). *Handling the young cerebral palsied child at home*. (2nd ed.) New York: E. P. Dulton.

Fisher, S., Painter, M., & Milmoe, G. (1981). Swallowing disorders in infancy. *Pediatric Clinics of North America, 28* (4), 845–853.

Frank, M., & Gatewood, O. (1966). Transient pharyngeal incoordination in the newborn. *American Journal of the Disabled Child, 3,* 178–181.

Gisel, E. (1991). Effect of food texture on the development of chewing between six months and two years of age. *Developmental Medicine and Child Neurology, 33,* 69–79.

Gryboski, J. (1965). The swallowing mechanism of the neonate: esophageal and gastric motility. *Pediatrics, 35* (1), 445–452.

Illingworth, R. (1964). The critical or sensitive period, with special references to certain feeding problems in infants and children. *Journal of Pediatrics, 65,* 839–848.

Illingworth, R. (1969). Sucking and swallowing difficulties in infancy: diagnostic problem of dysphagia. *Archives of Disabilities of Childhood, 44,* 655–664.

Kenny, D., Koheil, R., Greenberg, J., Reid, D., Milner, M., Eng, D., Moran, R., & Judd, P. (1989). Development of a multidisciplinary feeding profile for children who are dependent feeders. *Dysphagia, 4,* 16–28.

Kramer, S. (1989). Radiologic examination of the swallowing impaired child. *Dysphagia, 3,* 117–125.

Lanza, D., Koltai, P., Parnes, S., Decker, J., Wing, P., & Fortune, J. (1990). Predictive value of the glascow coma scale for tracheotomy in head-injured patients. *Annals of Otology Rhinology and Laryngology, 99,* 38–41.

Linden, P. & Siebens, A. (1983). Dysphagia: predicting laryngeal penetration. *Archives of Physical Medicine Rehabilitation, 64,* 281–283.

Logan, W., & Bosma, J. (1967). Oral and pharyngeal dysphagia in infancy. *Pediatric Clinics of North America, 14*(1), 47–59.

Loughlin, G. (1989). Respiratory consequences of swallowing and aspiration. *Dysphagia, 3,* 135–154.

Narayanan, I., Mehta, R., Choudhury, D., & Jain, B. (1991). Sucking on the "emptied" breast: Non-nutritive sucking with a difference. *Archives of Disease in Childhood, 66,* 241–244.

Nash, M. (1988). Swallowing problems in the tracheotomized patient. *Otolaryngologic Clinics of North America, 21* (4), 701–709.

Ramsay, M., & Zelazo, P. (1988). Food refusal in failure-to-thrive infants: nasogastric feeding combined with interactive-behavioral treatment. *Journal of Pediatric Psychology, 13*(3), 329–347.

Rogers, P., & Coleman, M. (1992). *Medical care in Down syndrome: A preventive medicine approach.* New York: Marcel Dekker.

Ryan, L., Ehrlich, S., & Finnegan, L. (1987). Cocaine abuse in pregnancy: Effects on the fetus and newborn. *Neurotoxicology and Teratology, 9,* 295–299.

Sasaki, C., Levine, P., Laitman, J., & Crelin, E. (1977). Postnatal descent of the epiglottis in man. *Archives of Otolaryngology, 103,* 169–171.

Sonies, B., & Baum, B. (1988). Evaluation of swallowing pathophysiology. *Otolaryngologic Clinics of North America, 21* (4), 637–648.

Staiano, A., Cucchiara, S., De-Vizia, B., Andreotti, M., & Auricchio, S. (1987). Disorders of upper esophageal sphincter motility in children. *Journal of Pediatric Gastroenterology and Nutrition, 6,* 892–898.

Steinscheinder, A., Weinstein, S., Diamond, E., (1982). The sudden infant death syndrome and apnea/obstruction during neonatal sleeping and feeding. *Pediatrics, 70,* 858–863.

Utinhl, T. (1966). Cricopharyngeal dysphagia in infancy. *Pediatrics, 43,* 402–406.

Vice, F., Heinz, J., Giuriati, G., Hood, M., & Bosma, J. (1990). Cervical auscultation of suckle feeding in newborn infants. *Developmental Medicine and Child Neurology, 32,* 760–768.

Westlake, H. & Rutherford, D. (1966). *Cleft palate.* Englewood Cliffs, NJ: Prentice-Hall.

Wolff, P. (1968). The serial organization of sucking in the young infant. *Pediatrics, 42* (6), 943–956.

Woolridge, M. (1986). The "anatomy" of infant sucking. *Midwifery, 2,* 164–171.

RIC Clinical Evaluation of Dysphagia: Pediatrics (CED—Pediatrics)

Wendy S. Perlin, MA, CCC-SLP
Maureen M. Boner, MS, CCC-SLP

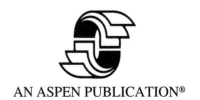

AN ASPEN PUBLICATION®

Name: _____

Case #:_____

Date of Birth: _____ Age: _____

Date of Evaluation: _____

Parent/Caregiver Questionnaire

Parent/Caregiver Interviewed: _____

1. In what position and seating system do you usually feed your child?

2. Are any special utensils or equipment used? (Please list)

3. Do you use any special feeding techniques? (Please list)

4. What are your child's likes and dislikes (foods, textures, temperatures)? (Please list)

5. What foods or beverages are difficult for your child to eat or drink? How so?

6. How long does it usually take to feed your child an average meal?

7. How much food does your child usually eat in one meal? (Describe an average meal.)

8. Do you supplement your child's oral diet in any way?

9. Has your child had any unusual problems with eating (e.g., reflux, food or liquid leaking from the nose)?

10. Was the introduction of solid foods difficult? How so?

11. Is there any history of allergies, asthma, or dietary restrictions?

12. Who usually feeds the child?

Name: _____   Date of Birth: _____   Age: _____

Case #: _____   Date of Evaluation: _____

Preassessment

BEHAVIOR
Age-appropriate:
Reduced attention:
Impulsivity:
Fatigue:
Agitation:
Manipulative behaviors (please list):

Other:

POSITIONING
Habitual feeding position:

Trial/optimal feeding position:

INTERFERING PATTERNS
Overall tone:
Primitive reflexes:

Abnormal patterns/posturing:

RESPIRATION
Within normal limits:
Raspy:
Labored:
Mouth-breather:
Other:

Clavicular:
Thoracic:
Abdominal:
Asthma:
Stridor:

FEEDING EQUIPMENT
Utensils (type and grip):

Cup (type):   Straw:

Bottle/nipple type:

Other:

TRACHEOSTOMY TUBE
Present:
Type:
Cuff:
One-way valve:
Frequency of suctioning:
Corking schedule:

Size:
Fenestrated:
Type:

ORAL INTAKE
Formula type:
Type of food eaten:
Amount per oral feeding:
    Liquid: _____ Solid: _____
Frequency of oral feedings:
    Liquid: _____ Solid: _____
Duration of average feeding:
History of intolerance:
    Type of food/liquid:
Other:

ALTERNATE FEEDING
Method of alternate feeding:
Supplemental formula:
Intake amount:
Time after last feeding:
Other:

MEDICAL CONTRAINDICATIONS
Fever: G-E reflux:
Tracheoesophageal fistula:
Tracheomalacia:
Other:

Rehabilitation Institute of Chicago CED—Pediatrics

Name: _____

Case #: _____

Date of Birth: _____

Date of Evaluation: _____

Age: _____

	Sensation (Right / Left)	Symmetry	Tone (Right / Left)	Related Features	Elicited — Individual or Repetitive	Range (L/R)	Rate (L/R)	Strength (L/R)	Coordination	Comments
FACE				Circle as appropriate or comment; Dysmorphic features:		L/R	L/R	L/R		
LIPS				Tremor; Retraction; Dysmorphic features:	Retraction; Protraction; Compression					
TONGUE				Tremor; Retraction; Bunched; Fasciculations; Short frenulum; Atrophy; Dysmorphic features:	Lateralization; Cheek pushes; Circular range of motion; Protrusion; Elevation outside lips; Elevation to hard palate; Depression					
DENTITION AND JAW				Good hygiene; Prosthesis; Missing teeth; Dental bite; Bruxism	Jaw opening					
PALATE				Arch: High / Flat / Normal; Cleft:; Type:						
VELO-PHARYNX	Gag ___ ; Hyper ___ ; Hypo ___			Tonsils:; Uvula:	Elevation on phonation; Nasality: WNL ___ Hypernasal ___ Hyponasal ___					
PHARYNX/ LARYNX					VOCAL QUALITY Clear ___ Wet ___ ; Laryngeal elevation on dry swallow: Present ___ Absent ___ Reduced ___	L R	L R	L R		

KEY: N = Normal/Symmetric; R = Reduced; E = Excessive; I = Irregular; D = Deviant/Asymmetric

The Pediatric Scale

Name: _____

Case #: _____

Date of Birth: _____ Age: ____

Date of Evaluation: _____

Age in Months:	0–3	4–6	7–9	10–12
Reflexes				
Rooting	P	A	A	A
Babkin	P	A	A	A
Palmomental	P	A	A	A
Transverse tongue	P	P	A	A
Bite	P	P	A	A
Gag	P	P	P	P
Startle	P	A	A	A
Grasp	P	A	A	A
ATNR	P	A	A	A
Face				
Varied facial expressions	A	P	P	P
Recognition of bottle/utensil	A	P	P	P
Anticipation of food/liquid	P*	P	P	P

	0–3	4–6	7–9			10–12		
	Bottle	Bottle	Bottle	Cup	Spoon/Fork	Bottle	Cup	Spoon/Fork
Lips								
Approximation	P	P	P	P	P	P	P	P
Active lip closure	A	P	P	P	P	P	P	P
Active lip movement	A	P	P	EM	EM	P	EM	P
Active pull on nipple	A	A	P			P		
Maintain lip closure	A	EM	P	EM	EM	P	EM	P
Liquid/food lost	P	A	A	P	P*	A	P*	A
Remove food from utensil					EM			P
Tongue								
Cupped configuration	P	P	A	A	A	A	A	A
Protrusion on swallow	P	A	A	P	P	A	P*	P
Lateralization					EM			P
Ability to form bolus		EM	P	EM	P	P	P	P
Good posterior movement of food/liquid	P	P	P	P	P	P	P	P
Ability to clean lips				A	A		EM	P
Dentition/Mandible								
Wide excursion	P	A	A	P	A	A	A	A
Good jaw control	A	P	P	A	EM	P	EM	P
Ability to bite off cookie					EM			P
Stability by biting on cup				P			P	
Vertical chew					P			P
Rotary chew					A			A
Ability to initiate and maintain chewing					P			P
Coordination								
Active suck	EM	P	P	EM	A	P	P	A
Active suckle	P	P	A	P	A	A	A	A
# Suck(le)s before breath	2–3	20	20+			20+		

Key: Present (**P**) Still present some of the time (**P***) Emerging skill (**EM**) Absent (**A**) Not applicable

Rehabilitation Institute of Chicago CED—Pediatrics

Copyright © 1994 by Aspen Publishers, Inc.

Name: _____

Case #: _____

Date of Birth: _____   Age: ____

Date of Evaluation: _____

Age in Months:	13–18			19–24			24+	
Reflexes								
Rooting	A			A			A	
Babkin	A			A			A	
Palmomental	A			A			A	
Transverse tongue	A			A			A	
Bite	A			A			A	
Gag	P			P			P	
Startle	A			A			A	
Grasp	A			A			A	
ATNR	A			A			A	
Face								
Varied facial expressions	P			P			P	
Recognition of bottle/utensil	P			P			P	
Anticipation of food/liquid	P			P			P	
	Bottle	Cup	Spoon/Fork	Bottle	Cup	Spoon/Fork	Cup	Spoon/Fork
Lips								
Approximation	P	P	P	P	P	P	P	P
Active lip closure	P	P	P	P	P	P	P	P
Active lip movement	P	P	P	P	P	P	P	P
Active pull on nipple	P			P				
Maintain lip closure	P	EM	P	P	P	P	P	P
Liquid/food lost	A	P*	A	A	A	A	A	A
Remove food from utensil			P			P		P
Tongue								
Cupped configuration	A	A	A	A	A	A	A	A
Protrusion on swallow	A	P*	A	A	A	A	A	A
Lateralization			P			P		P
Ability to form bolus	P	P	P	P	P	P	P	P
Good posterior movement of food/liquid	P	P	P	P	P	P	P	P
Ability to clean lips		P	P		P	P	P	P
Dentition/Mandible								
Wide excursion	A	A	A	A	A	A	A	A
Good jaw control	P	EM	P	P	P	P	P	P
Ability to bite off cookie			P			P		P
Stability by biting on cup		A			A		A	
Vertical chew			P*			A		A
Rotary chew			EM			P		P
Ability to initiate and maintain chewing			P			P		P
Coordination								
Active suck	P	P	A	P	P	A	P	A
Active suckle	A	A	A	A	A	A	A	A
# Suck(le)s before breath	20+			20+				

Key: Present (**P**)   Still present some of the time (**P***)   Emerging skill (**EM**)   Absent (**A**)   Not applicable

Name: _____ Date of Birth: _____ Age: ____

Case #: _____ Date of Evaluation: _____

Summary of Feeding and Swallowing Patterns

General Impressions: _____

Interaction: _____

Interfering Patterns and Behaviors: _____

	Thin Liquid	Thick Liquid	Pureed Food	Ground Food	Chopped Food	Regular Food	Comments
LIPS							
Lip retraction							
Lip pursing:							
Loss of liquid: (Unilateral: ____ Bilateral: ____)							
Loss of food: (Unilateral: ____ Bilateral: ____)							
Increased drooling: ____							
No Problems Exhibited: ____							
TONGUE							
Residue in oral cavity:							
Pooling:							
Food packed in palate:							
Pocketing (Location: _____):							
Tongue thrust:							
Tongue retraction:							
Oral transit times (No. of sec):							
No Problems Exhibited: ____							
DENTITION/MANDIBLE							
Jaw thrust:							
Tonic bite reflex (Trigger point: _____):							
Jaw clenching:							
Munching/vertical chew:							
Bruxism:							
No Problems Exhibited: ____							
SWALLOWING							
Delayed trigger of pharyngeal swallow (No. of sec):							
Absent trigger of pharyngeal swallow:							
Swallows per bolus (List number):							
Wet vocal quality before the swallow:							
Wet vocal quality after the swallow:							
Cough before swallow:							
Cough during swallow:							
Cough after swallow:							
Reduced laryngeal elevation:							
No Problems Exhibited: ____							

RESULTS
RECOMMENDATIONS

Rehabilitation Institute of Chicago CED—Pediatrics

Copyright © 1994 by Aspen Publishers, Inc.

◆ CHAPTER 5 ◆

Dysphagia: A Model for Differential Diagnosis for Adults and Children

Barbara C. Sonies

INTRODUCTION

Treatment of swallowing disorders has become the increasing responsibility and primary role of many speech-language pathologists employed in medical centers, clinics, nursing homes, special institutions, and home health and rehabilitation agencies. The ability to select the appropriate diagnostic tool has also become increasingly important in these settings because correct diagnosis of the source of swallowing difficulty is the basis for all subsequent types of treatment. Information gained from a careful feeding interview, especially in children, coupled with an observation of actual food intake, may provide sufficient data to develop a treatment plan without the use of any instrumental procedures. However, many times clinicians feel that they are providing inadequate service without conducting a "procedure." Also, children and adults are often administered the same set of test procedures regardless of their symptoms and regardless of inherent risks and dangers. When the longer-term bioeffects of these procedures are not carefully considered, the health of the individual may be compromised. Furthermore, many institutions and medical centers are under fiscal constraints to ensure that a prescribed intervention will produce the best results in the most cost-effective manner. Payers are looking for ways to ensure that a prescribed intervention will produce a positive outcome from a sound diagnostic base. To maximize dysphagia treatment outcomes, reduce bioeffects, and reduce the cost of health care of persons with difficulty swallowing, proper matching of the type, safety, and risks of different diagnostic techniques for dysphagia must be taken into consideration.

A differential diagnosis must take many factors into account that occur before, during, and after the diagnostic procedure. Differential diagnosis allows clinicians to match the results of the diagnosis to risks, as well as symptoms and age of each client and to ensure the most appropriate diagnostic package for each client. Proper selection and matching is the key to a diagnostic tool box.

This chapter presents some criteria, cautions, and models to allow clinicians to make the best possible diagnostic and follow-up evaluation choices for clients and to give options for flexibility in the decision-making process leading up to treatment. Because the cautions and needs of children and adults differ, basic guidelines for use of the different procedures in various developmental categories are suggested.

OVERVIEW OF TECHNIQUES

Whereas there are several diagnostic procedures for evaluation of swallowing disorders, many techniques that are readily available in medical/clinical settings may not be commonly used. The order of frequency of use of the diagnostic procedures for dysphagia are

- videofluoroscopy
- ultrasound
- fiberoptic endoscopy (FEES)
- manometry
- scintigraphy
- cervical auscultation (CA)

Table 5-1 briefly describes each of these procedures and provides references for more detailed descriptions of the use and development of each specific technique. Videofluorography is the most frequently used procedure for evaluation of swallowing in both adults and children and may be used exclusively by some practitioners. This is true for a variety of reasons, including

- ease of interpretation
- difficulty scheduling other procedures
- lack of staff training in other techniques
- precedents in particular settings that dictate use of fluorography

Because X-radiation is produced by videofluorography, it is imperative that clinicians use (or know when to recommend) other less harmful procedures, especially for children or infirm adults who are likely to be exposed to other radiographic procedures.

Table 5-1 Instrumental Procedures for Dysphagia: An Overview

Procedure	*Comments*
Videofluoroscopy (Logemann, 1983, 1986)	• permits observation of the oral preparatory, oral, pharyngeal, and esophageal aspects of the swallow, before, during, and after the event • provides a qualitative estimate of aspiration • requires the ingestion of barium-coated material • conducted by a speech-language pathologist and a radiography technician; video output should be analyzed by both a speech-language pathologist and a radiologist
Ultrasonography (Shawker, Sonies, & Stone, 1984; Sonies, 1991b; Sonies, Parent, Morrish, & Baum, 1988; Stone & Shawker, 1986)	• visualizes the oral cavity and hypopharynx during swallowing • any commercial ultrasound real-time sector or phased-array system is used • transducer is placed submentally below the chin to obtain image • conducted by a speech-language pathologist and an ultrasound technician
Fiberoptic Endoscopy (FEES) (Langmore, Schatz, & Olsen, 1988)	• examines laryngeal penetration and laryngeal functioning during swallowing • uses a flexible fiberoptic endoscope passed transnasally through the nasopharynx and hypopharynx and positioned in the laryngopharynx above the false vocal folds, superior to the epiglottis • images can be stored on tape if a video system is connected to the endoscopy equipment • performed by an otolaryngologist or a speech-language pathologist specially trained in its administration
Manometry (Castell, Dalton, & Castell, 1990; Dodds, Kahrilas, Dent, & Hogan, 1987; McConnel, Cerenko, Jackson, & Hersh, 1988)	• assesses pressure dynamics of the pharynx and upper esophageal sphincter during swallowing • requires the transnasal insertion of a catheter housing a series of intraluminal solid-state transducers, which record the changes in pressure resulting from swallowing • performed by a gastroenterologist

continues

Table 5-1 Instrumental Procedures for Dysphagia: An Overview (continued)

Procedure	Comments
Scintigraphy (Fleming, Muz, & Hamlet, 1990; Hamlet, Muz, Patterson, & Jones, 1989; Humphries et al., 1987)	• precisely quantifies volume of a bolus in any area at a particular time or over time • can quantify regurgitation and/or the amount of material aspirated into the tracheobronchial region • requires ingestion of a radioactive bolus • radioactivity of bolus is recorded as material passes through oral cavity, pharynx, and esophagus • requires expertise of a physician with training in nuclear medicine
Cervical Auscultation (CA) (Vice, Heinz, Giuriati, Hood, & Bosma, 1990)	• may detect the presence of a swallow and possible aspiration • stethoscope is placed against patient's neck during swallowing • clinician listens for the sound of a swallow and the characteristic sound of air mixing with liquids that suggests aspiration • performed by a speech-language pathologist

FACTORS IN DIFFERENTIAL DIAGNOSTICS OF DYSPHAGIA

The focus of this chapter is the use of instrumental techniques as a basis for the differential diagnosis. However, the reader is referred to Chapters 3 and 4 on the clinical examination that forms the basis for decision making. It is from a thorough history, interview, oropharyngeal sensorimotor examination, review of medical systems, medications, food preferences, and diet that one will form the primary diagnosis and determine the first level of the diagnosis decision pathway (Fig. 5-1).

To make a differential diagnosis of dysphagia, the examiner/clinician must take several factors into consideration (Fig. 5-1). The first factor requires knowledge of the *characteristics* of the type of image produced by the instrumental procedure so that the proper view of the oropharynx is obtained for each patient/client. At the next level, a set of *clinical selection factors* should be considered to evaluate the components of the swallow and of bolus transport provided with each procedure. Consideration of the ways that the procedure itself affects *patient safety* and comfort are made at the third level. Patient compliance is also considered at level 3; a dangerous or invasive procedure should not be performed if patient cooperation or health status is an issue. The final selection of the correct technique(s) is made at the fourth level using *client/symptom selection factors* to match the output of the technique to the symptoms and age of each patient. When all these levels are considered, the diagnostician will have sufficient information to choose the most appropriate procedure for each individual.

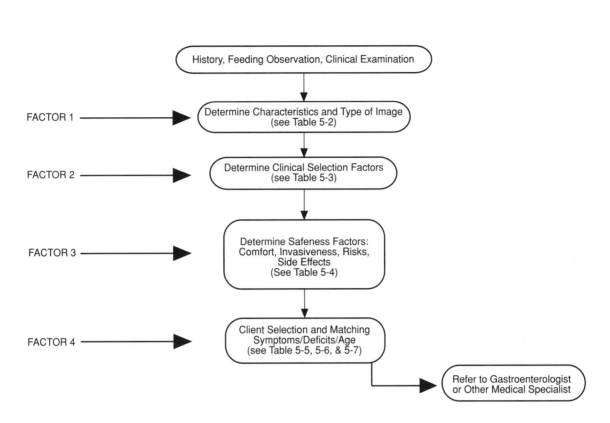

Figure 5-1 Diagnosis Decision Pathway: Factors 1 through 4

Factor 1: Characteristics and Type of Image

All dysphagia diagnostic techniques can be described by the *type* of image that each produces and whether each image is a complete or partial representation of the oropharyngeal swallow (see Table 5-2).

Complete versus Partial

Complete images are those that simultaneously present the anatomy of the swallow and the flow of the bolus through the aerodigestive system. The patient or the instrument may need to be manipulated or moved by the examiner to view the entire sequence of the bolus as it passes from the oral cavity into the esophagus. Videofluoroscopy provides a complete image in that the bony structures of the oropharynx, the airway, and the digestive tract can be seen at the same time that the bolus (impregnated with contrast material) moves through the system. Use of barium contrast material outlines the surface of the soft tissues of the palate, tongue, pharynx, larynx, and esophagus. Specific muscles cannot be seen, the soft tissue structures of the mouth are shadowed from view by the mandible, and the laryngeal structures may not be visible unless they are coated by aspirated mate-

Table 5-2 Factor 1: Characteristics and Types of Imaging Procedures

	Procedure/Technique					
Characteristics	Videofluoroscopy	Ultrasound	Fees	Scintigraphy	Manometry	Cervical Auscultation
Complete	+					
Partial		+	+ larynx	+	+	
Dynamic	+	+	+ with video	+	only bolus flow	acoustic
Static						
Pictorial	+	+		digitized bolus		
Point tracking					+	with microphone
Observational			without video			+
Multiple plane	+	+				
Single plane			transverse	sagittal/ frontal	sagittal	

+ indicates characteristic is present

rial. However, videofluoroscopy is easy to interpret as the images produce a clear likeness to the actual anatomy.

All the other procedures used in the diagnosis of dysphagia can be called incomplete because they do not depict a complete view of the anatomy simultaneously with bolus motion. Ultrasound clearly visualizes the muscles, depicts the surfaces between muscles, organs, and blood vessels, distinguishes tumors, masses, air, liquids, facial borders, and normal tissues, and simultaneously demonstrates motion. Ultrasound does not, however, depict bone. The examiner must move the transducer to visualize the anatomy as it produces a tomograph or pictured slice of the anatomy at several anatomic planes. Although the FEES produces a clear view of a single segment of the anatomy in a single transverse plane, the view is impeded when the larynx adducts, the pharynx constricts, and/or the epiglottis lowers during the swallow. Scintigraphy produces a digitized image of the flow of the bolus but does not display actual structures. Simulated anatomic areas are produced for scintigraphy using computer processing. Manometry, by itself, produces an analog time display of pressure changes associated with bolus flow through the pharynx into the esophagus without any anatomic referents. Manometry may be paired with other procedures such as videofluoroscopy to add a pictorial display of the anatomy. Cervical auscultation produces no image and is an auditory-tactile observational technique that associates sound picked up by a stethoscope with bolus passage through the pharynx.

Static versus Dynamic

Other considerations regarding the type of image are whether the image is *static* or *dynamic*. Because swallowing is a dynamic process that occurs rapidly and in sequence, rarely does one use a static procedure for evaluation. In the case in which there is suspicion of a bony obstruction or a soft tissue mass causing the difficulty swallowing, a static radiograph or a computed tomography (CT) scan would be recommended for differential diagnosis. When used alone without video taping, the FEES is a static endoscopic technique that is used to view the anatomy of the vocal folds. By video taping the study, the entire procedure is stored, showing the dynamic aspects of laryngeal function and airway protection.

Pictorial versus Point Tracking versus Observational

In most cases, images are easier to interpret when they are *pictorial* in that the normal anatomy in its actual form, density, and/or proportions are seen. Videofluoroscopy, ultrasound, CT, and magnetic resonance imaging (MRI) are pictorial. Techniques that track points or movements, as on an oscilloscope (e.g., manometry or research procedures such as electromyogram (EMG) and electroglottogram (EGG)), can be used to provide quantitative information regarding amplitude, direction, force of movement, or degree or type of muscle contractions and to chart simultaneous respiratory activity. Point tracking systems are usually coupled with a pictorial system and may be used for research purposes (Stone & Shawker, 1986). Observational procedures involve no storage or collection of data but examine an activity or behavior immediately and directly as it occurs. The observational output from CA can be converted into a point tracking system if a contact microphone is attached to the neck and the output displayed on an oscilloscope.

Multiple versus Single Plane

Because different components of the swallow can be studied from *multiple planes* it is important to select the views or planes to be visualized during a procedure (Fig. 5-2). The side (sagittal, lateral) view in the midline plane is best obtained on videofluorography or ultrasound. Sagittal views provide essential information regarding the tongue, velum, epiglottis, hyoid, pharynx, and flow of the bolus. Also, a sagittal view can indicate any unusual patterns of timing and incoordination (e.g., tremors, spasms, contractions, fasciculations) of the oropharyngeal muscles. Measurements of the transport and timing of the bolus through the oropharynx are best taken in the sagittal plane because the entire swallow can be seen. Radiograph, ultrasound, and scintigraphic studies can all be performed in multiple planes (i.e., sagittal, parasagittal, transverse, frontal, coronal) by moving the position of the individual or the scanner. The ability to view the swallow from different positions has proven to be quite informative. In stroke cases or head trauma with hemiparesis, pharyngeal asymmetry and pooling is best seen on fluoroscopy; lingual paresis is best seen on ultrasound. Asymmetries causing delays in bolus transport and/or pharyngeal pooling can be seen on the frontal anteroposterior (A/P) view, whereas epiglottal lowering and velar elevation can be seen in the fluorographic sagittal view. An off-midline or parasagittal view of the tongue or hypopharynx may provide information useful for treatment in cases with hemiparesis or unilateral weakness. Different aspects of tongue motion are detected from sagittal and coronal views on ultrasound. Tongue asymmetries and compensatory or unusual movements of the floor of the mouth can be viewed in the coronal plane and sagittal plane with ultrasound. These findings can be used to assist the patient in correct bolus placement and oral preparation maneuvers and to provide feedback during treatment. Hyoid bone motion and extra lingual gestures that do not lead to a complete swallow are seen in the sagittal ultrasound plane. Aspiration as well as laryngeal penetration can be seen on both sagittal and frontal views of the laryngopharynx with videofluorography, and residue after a swallow is seen on the transverse view provided by FEES. Adduction or abduction of the larynx is also noted in the transverse view with FEES and the A/P view in videofluorography.

Based solely on the decision of what level of completeness is desired and how many planes need to be evaluated, a first-factor decision regarding selection of a technique can be made. Table 5-2 lists each technique and the factor 1 characteristics that are associated with each procedure. Under only the most unusual circumstances should a static, observational, or point tracking procedure be used alone. In other words, the instrumental procedure chosen will be most useful if it is dynamic and complete. However, this suggestion is tempered with the considerations that will need to be made at the second and third factor levels regarding clinical selection and safety.

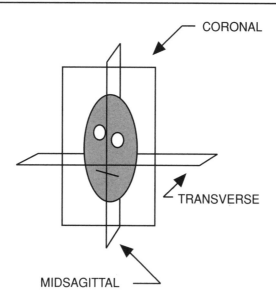

Fig. 5-2 Simplified Schematic of Imaging Planes

Factor 2: Clinical Selection Factors

In making *clinical selection* decisions regarding which procedure(s) should be used, several factors should be given primary consideration. They are

- ability to visualize and track both the bolus and the motions of the swallowing mechanism in real-time
- ability to detect entry of the bolus into the airway
- ease of using natural food
- whether the procedure itself can be used in treatment and for follow-up

The set of clinical selection factors is displayed on Table 5-3. Each factor is listed in columns at the top of the table with the diagnostic procedures/techniques listed in descending order beneath them (i.e., the best diagnostic technique for that factor is listed at the top of each column).

Visualization

The factor listed in the first column is *visualization of the swallow*. When the complete oropharyngeal swallow is displayed, diagnosing the physiologic and temporospatial components of dysphagia is facilitated. One should be able to visualize bolus preparation and tongue motion before the swallow, oral and pharyngeal bolus transport, hyolaryngeal elevation, velar and epiglottal motion, and bolus passage through the esophagus. The only technique that depicts the entire sequence of activity is videofluoroscopy. Although the esophagus is not visible, the entire oropharyngeal swallow is depicted on ultrasound imaging. This is because the fulcrum of swallow motion is the hyoid bone. The hyoid moves from rest to an upward-forward position under the mandible at the start of the swallow. Hyoid elevation serves to elevate the larynx and lower the epiglottis as the bolus flows through the pharynx. Because the hyoid remains elevated when the bolus passes through the pharynx and returns to its resting position only when the bolus has entered the cervical esophagus, the duration of the entire oropharyngeal swallow is captured on ultrasound (Sonies et al., 1988). Recent work in progress using simultaneous ultrasound/videofluoroscopy has confirmed this finding (Sonies & Cordaro, 1992). Ultrasound imaging cannot demarcate the bolus after it has passed into the hypopharynx and cannot track the bolus as it moves into the esophagus. The larynx can be seen on ultrasound from the transverse view using another of the scanning transducers.

Similarly, the bolus cannot be tracked as it moves from the oral cavity through the pharynx with FEES, as endoscopy can only be used to detect laryngeal penetration and residue in the valleculae, vocal folds, and pyriform sinuses after the swallow. The actual moment when the swallow occurs is not seen with FEES. Neither the anatomy nor the motion of anatomic structures is seen on scintigraphy; however, it is a procedure that gives complete information on bolus transport from the oral cavity to the esophagus. Scintigraphy is a technique that can indicate whether the bolus has entered the tracheobronchial tree (still radiographs can be used to see tracheal or lung infiltration) and is the only technique that presently has programs to quantify bolus volume. Manometry gives

Table 5-3 Factor 2: Clinical Selection Factors

Visualizes Complete Swallow: Anatomy (A), Bolus Transport (B)	Detects Aspiration (A) or Laryngeal Penetration (LP)	Uses Natural Diets	Use During Treatment
Best	*Best*	*Best*	*Best*
Videofluoroscopy (A & B)	Scintigraphy (A & LP) Videofluoroscopy (A & LP)	Ultrasound Cervical auscultation	Ultrasound
Partial	*Partial*	*Partial*	*Moderate*
Ultrasound (A & B—partial) FEES (A & B—partial) Scintigraphy (B) Manometry (B)	Manometry (reflux) FEES (LP) Cervical auscultation (LP?)	FEES (food coloring)	FEES Cervical auscultation
Unable to Visualize	*Minimal*	*Minimal*	*Minimal*
Cervical auscultation	Ultrasound (LP?)	Videofluoroscopy (barium-coated) Scintigraphy	Videofluoroscopy Scintigraphy

information on the timing and the flow of the bolus from the pharynx through the esophagus but does not display the swallow or the actual anatomy. Cervical auscultation, when used by a trained clinician, may provide auditory information that can be associated with the transport of the bolus through the pharynx (Vice et al., 1990).

Aspiration

The ability to detect *aspiration* is a primary reason for conducting a swallowing examination. Any additional evidence of laryngeal penetration before, during, or after the swallow is a negative sign and, when observed, serves as a diagnostic alert for the clinician. From examining column 2 on Table 5-3, we can see that scintigraphy is the best technique for detecting aspiration, followed closely by videofluoroscopy. Whereas videofluoroscopy shows aspiration and laryngeal penetration during the actual study, scintigraphic studies are interpreted from computerized displays of bolus flow and can be made at the time of the swallow or at any later interval. Volumetric measures of the amount of bolus remaining in each area can be displayed over any time period. Because radioactivity of ingested material is quantified, scintigraphy can be used to detect accumulation of bolus material in the lungs after the swallow.

Manometric studies do not detect aspiration but allow reflux activity to be measured by quantifying pressure changes that occur after the swallow in the esophagus. The FEES is an excellent technique for detecting bolus material remaining in the laryngeal vestibule and in the pyriform sinuses. By adding food coloring, material remaining in the laryngopharynx after the swallow will be visible using the scope. Although aspiration is not directly detected on ultrasound of the oral cavity, transverse laryngeal ultrasound imaging may be able to detect residue in the pyriform sinuses in a manner similar to FEES (Sonies, 1991b).

Selection of Foods

Use of natural diets or favorite foods is suggested when studying the swallow of patients who are infirm, uncooperative, or demented or for infants and children who refuse barium. Ultrasound and cervical auscultation are not dependent on contrast material during a study, and thus any food and all textures and consistencies can be used. In any case, if the technique uses radiation, caution should be exercised in relation to length of exposure when conducting studies using a wide variety of foods.

Applicable in Treatment

The primary reason to perform any diagnostic technique is to demonstrate the deficits or main symptoms that produce difficulty swallowing. An additional advantage of selecting a technique is whether it can be used to demonstrate to the patient how changes in different movements or positions can facilitate safer swallowing (i.e., in treatment). Ultrasound is the only technique that can be used with total safety to visualize therapeutic modifications and all alterations in the oropharyngeal swallow during treatment. Because ultrasound is free of bioeffects, it can be used as a biofeedback system during treatment. Furthermore, it can be used repeatedly, under different treatment conditions and for long periods of time with a wide variety of foods and postures. The movements and positions of the head, tongue, bolus, floor muscles, and hyoid can be altered and monitored during bolus placement and bolus transport. The effects of different food textures can be easily demonstrated to the patient. The patient can match correct and incorrect oral activity and use prerecorded videotaped samples as models. The other procedures are of limited-to-minimal use during treatment because their output is not representational and/or because of safety considerations.

Factor 3: Safeness Factors

Because many clinicians conduct follow-up evaluations of swallowing to confirm results of treatment and to follow progression of disease, they must make decisions regarding the *risks, side effects, comfort,* and *invasiveness* of procedures. These decisions should be made at the initial intake when the first evaluation is being conducted. In other words, the examiner should consider which follow-up procedures will be used and plan for the safeness factors at this time.

Risks

The main risk to the client is the long-term effect of irradiation. Because most persons will have many radiographs taken over their lifetimes and because of the cumulative effects of dental procedures, routine chest radiographs, mammography, and radiographs to detect breaks in bones, the dysphagia examination cannot be considered as a single exposure. Videofluorographic equipment should be calibrated yearly for radiation and adjusted as needed. There are guidelines for radiation exposure (e.g., 3 rem to a tissue in 13 weeks and 5 rem/year; for children, this is lowered by 10 percent—NIH Guidelines [see Sonies, 1991a]).

Table 5-4 depicts, in descending order, the irradiation risk posed by each procedure. Although there is no radiation risk with FEES or manometry, there is the possibility that tissue damage, nose bleeding, or apnea could result from nasopharyngeal insertion of the endoscope. There also is a slight chance that the anesthetic could produce a topical reaction or induce choking or gagging. There are no known risks resulting from using real-time ultrasound or from applying a stethoscope to the neck.

Side Effects

Side effects can be immediate or result from long-term use of a procedure. For example, the side effects of irradiation may not show up until years after exposure when tissues exhibit necrosis or wasting or when vascular changes are noted. Irradiation can shrink salivary gland tissue, which will reduce salivation and alter mucus formation and thus make swallowing more difficult. Insertion of a nasoendoscope may result in adverse reactions such as perforation of the oronasopharyngeal mucosa and bleeding or laryngospasm. Some people have an allergic reaction to topical anesthetics, and the elderly individual may react negatively or exhibit breathing difficulty or cardiac arrhythmia. Infants and children must be treated with caution, especially with any procedure that has irradiation,

Table 5-4 Factor 3: Safeness Factors

	Risks (e.g., Radiation)	Side Effects	Invasiveness	Comfort
Most	Videofluoroscopy Manofluorography	FEES	Manometry	Ultrasound CA Videofluoroscopy
↓	Scintigraphy	Manometry Manofluorography	FEES	
	FEES Manometry	Scintigraphy Videofluoroscopy	Videofluoroscopy Scintigraphy	Scintigraphy
↓ Least	CA Ultrasound	CA Ultrasound	CA Ultrasound	FEES Manometry

and should not have multiple or serial radiographs unless absolutely necessary. Ultrasound imaging is the only procedure that is without any known side effects and can be used for infants and children as often as needed to monitor change.

Invasiveness

Any procedure that has potential for bruising or causing lesions or perforation of the skin, mucosa, and tissues is considered invasive. Application of a fixative or glue to the skin to stabilize a piece of equipment can be invasive. If the procedure causes the individual to feel pain because of pressure or puncture, it can be considered invasive. Also, the long-term change in a tissue or organ can be considered invasive. Most of the procedures used to diagnose dysphagia have some degree of invasiveness; manometry and the fiberoptic endoscope are most invasive because they require anesthetics and insertion of a tube into the nasopharynx. Videofluorography and scintigraphy are minimally invasive because contrast material must be ingested; this is considered unpleasant to a few persons who may react by retching.

Comfort

When choosing a procedure, the aspect of patient comfort is usually not given priority. However, for individuals who have swallowing difficulty, an uncomfortable examination may produce artifacts that can be confused with symptoms of dysphagia. Consider the effects of placing the patient in a position in which the neck is hyperextended or the shoulders rounded and head protruded; these positions may be so uncomfortable that the patient cannot swallow in a normal fashion. Some people react adversely to being in an enclosed space or to having anything touching their bodies. If an examination room is too cold, hot or not well ventilated, it may cause episodes of light-headedness or sweating, thus making the examination unreliable.

Any instrumental procedures may cause anxiety for some patients, but in general, ultrasound and cervical auscultation pose no discomfort and the patient can be placed in any viewing position. For a few obese patients, the fluoroscopic unit is too small or the chair may be difficult for them to stabilize. Procedures that require intubation may cause some discomfort and are listed in Table 5-4. To best understand the implications of this table, consider the example of ultrasound imaging, which is the most comfortable, least invasive technique with the least risks and the fewest side effects.

Factor 4: Client/Symptom Selection and Matching

The end stage of the diagnostic decision pathway is to match the symptoms displayed during feeding observations and the clinical examination with the individual patient's complaints and needs. At this stage, the age of the patients and their medical, surgical, and cognitive function should be factored into the selection process. One must always refer back to the preceding three levels and consider the following parameters:

- the correct viewing plane(s)
- the safety and comfort of the procedure
- whether this is the first evaluation or a follow-up
- need for repeated studies to track progression of disease, recovery, or effects of treatment
- whether the study will focus on safety of oral feeding or bolus transport

If the person is cognitively intact and can follow directions, the next step is to consider the symptoms and main complaints, pair the patient with the technique suggested for a specific condition, and then consider the age of the individual. If it is apparent that the oropharyngeal stage is normal but esophageal transport appears abnormal, the clinician must refer the patient to a gastroenterologist or other physician for a definitive diagnosis.

Matching

The main complaints or symptoms of dysphagia are listed on Table 5-5 and are matched with the most appropriate technique(s) for that symptom. Also, conditions associated with dysphagia are paired with the technique most likely to assess the dysphagic complications of that condition (Table 5-6).

If the main complaint is indicative of respiratory difficulty or suggests likelihood of aspiration or laryngeal penetration, videofluoroscopy is indicated. If aspiration has been noted, scintigraphy can

Table 5-5 Factor 4: Matching Complaint or Symptom to the Technique

Complaint Clusters	Techniques	Comments
Respiratory difficulty Choking Gagging Hoarse voice after drinking Gurgling sounds	→ Videofluoroscopy Scintigraphy FEES Cervical auscultation	Possible aspiration Pooling and laryngeal penetration: consult ENT
Problems with solids Painful swallowing Feeling a lump Food catches in throat Weight loss	→ CT MRI Videofluoroscopy	Signs of possible mass or obstruction: check with M.D.
Difficulty chewing Oral dryness	→ Ultrasound	Can be due to medications, oral infections, effects of chemotherapy
Altered taste Changed food preferences	→ None needed if no other complaint	
Difficulty with pills Slow eater Difficulty with liquids	→ Ultrasound Videofluoroscopy	Indicates possible neurologic problem
Heartburn Indigestion Reflux	→ Manometry	Refer to M.D.: locus in esophagus or gastrointestinal tract

be used to determine whether there is infiltration into the tracheobronchial tree or the lungs. A static chest radiograph is often used to determine if there is lung damage and cystic or other tissue changes.

Complaints such as painful swallowing, feeling of a lump in the throat, food catching, and rapid weight loss may be signs of tumors or masses and require radiograph procedures such as CT, MRI, or videofluoroscopy. A hoarse gurgling voice indicates pooling in the pyriform sinus or on the ventricular folds and should be confirmed by use of videofluoroscopy or FEES. If no other technique is available and the patient cannot be moved (e.g., with infirm elderly or comatose patients), cervical auscultation can be used. Difficulty chewing, oral dryness, excessive mucus, and other complaints of this nature suggest that the underlying cause may be medications, oral infections, or the after-effects of chemotherapy or radiation. There are a variety of immunologic conditions such as Sjogren's disease or Sicca syndrome that produce these oral symptoms. To diagnose these complaints, a noninvasive technique, such as ultrasound, is recommended to examine the oral and oral preparatory stages. Alterations in taste and changes in food preference are not usually suggestive of dysphagia and do not require instrumental diagnosis if they are the only symptoms. Changes in taste and food preferences may be related to normal aging and the variety of medications the person is taking. In some rare instances, a tumor or systemic disease may be the cause. When the individual complains of difficulty swallowing pills, that eating has slowed, and of difficulty with liquids, the underlying cause could be neurologic. In this case, the complaint should be investigated further by both ultrasound and videofluoroscopy. Results of the baseline ultrasound study can then be used in later comparative studies. When heartburn, indigestion, and excessive reflux are main complaints, the patient should be referred to a physician, as the difficulty is most likely in the esophagus or the gastrointestinal tract. The physician may suggest an esophageal study or manometry or give medication for the reflux.

Videofluoroscopy should be used to diagnose neurologic and neuromotor conditions in adults. Table 5-6 lists specific medical conditions with the recommended technique for assessment of

Table 5-6 Factor 4: Matching Deficits to the Technique

Conditions	Techniques

Neuromuscular/Neurologic
  Amyotrophic lateral sclerosis
  Multiple sclerosis
  Parkinson's disease
  Huntington's disease
  Progressive supranuclear palsy
  Shy Drager syndrome
	Videofluoroscopy for initial examination
	Ultrasound or FEES for follow-up

Head and neck surgery	Ultrasound, videofluoroscopy, FEES
Stroke	Videofluoroscopy, ultrasound
Head injury or trauma	Videofluoroscopy, ultrasound, FEES
Comatose or in Intensive Care Unit	Cervical auscultation, ultrasound, observation
Dementias	Ultrasound, feeding observation

oropharyngeal swallowing. In most cases, an initial evaluation includes the videofluoroscopic evaluation and other less invasive procedures such as ultrasound or endoscopy for follow-up. At the National Institutes of Health (NIH), both videofluoroscopy and ultrasound are performed at the intake evaluation for comparison and the less invasive procedure is used for follow-up to reduce risks. If aspiration remains a symptom, a videofluoroscopic evaluation will be performed at follow-up. For comatose patients or those who are on respiratory support systems, oral reflexes are generally observed at bedside. Cervical auscultation is used for comatose patients in some facilities that focus on emergency medicine. It is generally unnecessary to expose elderly, infirm patients or those whose dysfunction is related to dementia, to X-radiation for a diagnosis regarding the safety of oral feeding. A history of pneumonia, lack of alertness, gurgling in the pharynx, raspy breathing, and reduced oral motor responses all signal that oral feeding is unsafe. Table 5-6 lists the recommended procedures for these patients.

Diagnosis and treatment of children with feeding difficulty is covered in detail elsewhere in this book. In this chapter, a brief discussion of diagnostic techniques for children follows. It is the firm opinion of the author that children should not be exposed to radiographic techniques unless it is absolutely necessary. Most children can be adequately evaluated by a developmental feeding evaluation and observation of their postural behaviors along with a complete diagnostic feeding interview with the parents or caretakers as described in Chapter 4. The main symptoms displayed by infants and children with feeding and swallowing difficulty are listed in Table 5-7 along with comments regarding which technique is suggested. It is in the best interest of the child that when he or she is failing to thrive or at high risk for aspiration, the diagnostic decision be made by the pediatrician and gastroenterologist in concert with the speech-language pathologist. For many children, an observation of oral-motor behavior is sufficient to begin treatment. Most children with feeding and swallowing difficulty have poor head, neck, jaw, and body control and abnormal muscle tone throughout the body. They often have tongue weakness, poor lip seal, impaired and weak sucking responses, incoordination of respiration and swallowing, and drooling along with nutritional imbalance. These children need to be placed in a program including intense oral-sensorimotor stimulation, positioning, and prefeeding exercises. These children need to learn how to synchronize swallowing and respiratory behaviors correctly. For most dysphagic children, oral stimulation and indirect feeding treatment programs should be initiated even though they are intubated. These are further discussed in Chapter 7.

Infants and children who have delayed development or slowed responses can be studied safely with ultrasound because it poses no risks even after lengthy or repeated studies. It is capricious to expose infants and children to radiation unless they are in respiratory distress or at risk for aspiration.

SUMMARY

A four-level model for selection of an appropriate procedure or technique has been presented as a guide to use in clinical decisions regarding diagnosis of dysphagia in infants, children, and adults.

Table 5-7 Factor 4: Matching Age and Symptom to the Technique

Symptoms	Techniques	Comments
Infant/Child		
Rales in chest with difficulty breathing	Refer to physician	Pulmonary consult
Developmental delays	None needed	Do oral examination
Failure to thrive	Refer to physician	Do oral examination Tube feeding
Poor body tone or posture Primitive oral reflexes Poor head, neck, jaw control	No instrumental technique needed	Sensory-motor stimulation and postural control
Oral-tactile defensiveness	No instrumental technique needed	Oral stimulation
Regurgitation	Refer to gastroenterologist	May require tube feeding or surgical procedure
Weak suck/suckle	Ultrasound	Oral stimulation
Craniofacial anomalies	Ultrasound	Check palate Oral examination ENT referral Refer to pediatrician
Aspiration, gurgling sounds on inhalation or phonation Pneumonia	Videofluoroscopy	May require alteration of food textures and position
Elderly—Infirm		
Bedridden Fragile Inattentive	Ultrasound Cervical auscultation FEES	Transportation and remuneration problems need consideration

This model is unique in that it guides the examiner to incorporate

- selection criterion on the types of images produced by each diagnostic procedure
- salient clinical selection factors
- safeness
- symptoms or complaints of the individual in the diagnostic decision

Consideration of which technique will be used at follow-up and which techniques can be used in treatment is also stressed. Because of inherent risks associated with irradiation, several instrumental techniques are presented to guide the examiner in the selection process. The age of the individual is a factor in some studies, and it is strongly suggested that caution be taken in evaluating children. Infants and children can usually be diagnosed from presenting symptoms coupled with a thorough feeding and oral sensorimotor developmental examination.

REFERENCES

Castell, J.A., Dalton, C.B., & Castell, D.D. (1990). Pharyngeal and upper esophageal sphincter manometry in humans. *American Journal of Physiology, 258,* 173–178.

Dodds, W.J., Kahrilas, P.J., Dent, J., & Hogan, W.J. (1987). Considerations about pharyngeal manometry. *Dysphagia, 1,* 209–214.

Fleming, S.M., Muz, J., & Hamlet, S. (1990). Practical scintigraphic application for dysphagic patient. *ASHA, 32,* 72.

Hamlet, S.L., Muz, J., Patterson, R., & Jones, L. (1989). Pharyngeal transit time: Assessment with videofluoroscopic and scintigraphic techniques. *Dysphagia, 4,* 4–15.

Humphries, B., Mathog, R., Miller, P., Rosen, R., Muz, J., & Nelson, R. (1987). Videofluoroscopic and scintigraphic analysis of dysphagia in the head and neck cancer patients. *Laryngoscope, 97,* 25–32.

Langmore, S.E., Schatz, K., & Olsen, N. (1988). Fiberoptic endoscopic examination of swallowing safety: A new procedure. *Dysphagia, 2,* 209–215.

Logemann, J.A. (1983). *Evaluation of swallowing disorders.* San Diego, CA: College-Hill Press.

Logemann, J.A. (1986). *Manual for the videofluorographic study of swallowing.* San Diego, CA: College-Hill Press.

McConnel, F.M.S., Cerenko, D., Jackson, R.T., & Hersh, T. (1988). Clinical application of manofluorogram. *Laryngoscope, 98,* 1–7.

Shawker, T.H., Sonies, B.C., & Stone, M. (1984). Sonography of speech and swallowing. In R.C. Saunders & M. Hill (Eds.), *Ultrasound annual* (pp. 237–260). New York: Raven Press.

Sonies, B.C. (1991a). Instrumental procedures for dysphagia diagnosis. *Swallowing Disorders: Seminars in Speech and Language, 12* (3), 185–198.

Sonies, B.C. (1991b). Ultrasound imaging and swallowing. In M. Donner & B. Jones (Eds.), *Normal and abnormal swallowing: Imaging in diagnosis and therapy* (pp. 109–119). New York: Springer.

Sonies, B.C., & Cordaro, M. (1992). *Image processing and instrumentation to compare hyoid bone motion from simultaneously recorded ultrasound and videofluorographic imaging of swallowing.* Poster presented at NIH Research Festival, Bethesda, Maryland.

Sonies, B.C., Parent, L.J., Morrish, K., & Baum, B.J. (1988). Evaluation of swallowing pathophysiology. *Otolaryngologic Clinics of North America, 21,* 638–648.

Stone, M., & Shawker, T. (1986). An ultrasound examination of tongue movement during swallowing. *Dysphagia, 1,* 78–83.

Vice, F.L., Heinz, J.M., Giuriati, G., Hood, M., and Bosma, J.F. (1990). Cervical auscultation of suckle feeding in newborn infants. *Developmental Medicine and Child Neurology, 32,* 760–768.

◆ CHAPTER 6 ◆

Treatment of Dysphagia in Adults

Bonnie J.W. Martin

INTRODUCTION

The clinical approach to the management of dysphagia must be based on an understanding of the physiologic and biomechanic properties of normal deglutition and on the systematic identification of deviations from these normal patterns. Through clinical and videofluorographic interpretation, a component-by-component analysis of the oral, pharyngeal, laryngeal, and cervical esophageal swallow dynamics is completed. Treatment techniques are then applied to the impaired mechanisms in a systematic manner.

Although the traditional segmentation of the swallow into phases or stages has descriptive use, it is important to remember that the phases of swallowing are arbitrary and overlap. The swallowing clinician rarely treats one component in isolation. Furthermore, a treatment applied to one structure usually facilitates improvement in other areas of the upper aerodigestive tract. An example is the propulsive mechanism of the tongue. Although the main goal may be improved strength and range of the tongue for more efficient oral bolus transport, the improved strength may improve pharyngeal clearance by increasing the range and strength of tongue base retraction and may also enhance speech production. Similarly, increasing the frequency of dry swallows may be a treatment goal directed toward improved management of accumulated oral secretions, but the repetitive dry swallows may also simultaneously strengthen pharyngeal muscle contraction (Martin, Nitschke, Schleicher, Chachere, & Dodds, 1992; Perlman, Luschei, & Du Mond, 1989).

Besides focusing on the swallowing mechanism, attention to the whole body health of the individual is warranted when contemplating treatment efficacy and planning treatment strategies. For example, consideration must be given to the cognitive function of the dysphagic patient, not only as it relates to swallow dysfunction but as it affects the patient's ability to carry out rehabilitation strategies (Martin & Corlew, 1990). Also, there is some clinical evidence that suggests sequential swallowing during mealtime produces changes in heart rate in some individuals (Martin et al., 1992). Although this potential physiologic effect may be functionally insignificant in otherwise healthy individuals, variations in heart rate may significantly affect swallowing in dysphagic patients with cardiac impairment. Because deglutition involves multisystem responses, all systems must be taken into account when treating the dysphagic patient.

Swallowing clinicians should also consider the effect of their dysphagia treatments on the function of the respiratory system (Martin, 1991, Martin, Logemann, Shaker, & Dodds, 1993; Martin et al., 1992) because there is increasing clinical and experimental evidence to support and delineate the neurophysiologic, structural, and functional interdependence between respiration and swallowing (Clark, 1920; Doty, 1968; Doty, Richmond, & Storey, 1967; Doty, 1968; Hukuhana & Okada, 1956; Martin, 1991; Miller, 1982; Nishino, Yonezawa, & Honda, 1985; Selley, Flack, Ellis, & Brooks, 1989a; Smith, Wolkove, Colacone, & Kreisman, 1989; Sumi, 1963; Wilson, Thach, Brouillette, & Abu-Osba, 1981). Swallowing may be considered an important respiratory defense mechanism (Martin, Corlew, Kirmani, & Olson, in press). It clears the pharynx of aspirated particles expectorated from the upper airways and often prevents the aspiration of refluxed gastric contents from the esophagus into the pharynx (Kennedy & Kent, 1985; Miller, 1982; Storey, 1976). Similarly, the aspiration of nasal and oral secretions that enter the pharynx and larynx is prevented by the functional swallow in healthy individuals. In the patient with coexisting respiratory and swallowing impairments, the work of breathing and swallowing may far exceed that which is characteristic of healthy adults and compromise swallow safety, oral nutrition, and hydration.

INDIRECT VERSUS DIRECT DYSPHAGIA MANAGEMENT

During the clinical and radiographic testing and analysis of the patient's swallowing mechanism, the clinician begins a problem-solving process regarding management. The initial question that must be answered is whether to manage the patient's dysphagia directly or indirectly, and several factors enter into this critical decision. Indirect management does not involve direct hands-on patient contact but includes recommendations given to caregivers by the swallowing clinician. Direct management, however, refers to routine rehabilitative practices with the patient. It may include the therapeutic administration of liquid or food stimuli or, if the patient is unable to tolerate oral intake safely, the implementation of rehabilitative methods without liquid or food substances.

The decision whether to manage a patient's dysphagia directly or indirectly depends on the nature and severity of the swallowing impairment, the etiology of the disorder, and the patient's prognosis for improvement. Direct management should be considered only if it is likely to make a difference in the quality of the patient's life, nutritional status, or safety. Third-party reimbursement requires the establishment of realistic and measurable goals and positive prognostic indicators for achievement of these goals. If these requirements cannot be met, direct dysphagia management is contraindicated. The patient's level of alertness, communicative and cognitive status, medical stability, endurance, and pulmonary function all play a role in the clinician's decision to manage the patient's dysphagia directly through routine therapy practices or indirectly through education or feeding adaptations suggested to caregivers and interdisciplinary team members.

INDIRECT MANAGEMENT

The term *indirect* does not connote unimportance. Rather, indirect management often plays a critical role in the total care of the dysphagic patient, particularly when direct intervention is not efficacious. For example, patients may suffer from end-stage progressive disease or have severe cognitive impairment that precludes the ability to follow even simple commands that are required for swallow rehabilitation (Curran & Groher, 1990; Mirro & Patey, 1991). Recommendations for tube feedings or food and liquid texture modifications represent methods of indirect dysphagia management (Curran, 1990).

It is not uncommon for patients to be able to swallow safely during videofluoroscopy, but their functional skills at the bedside may differ considerably because of problems with endurance, insight, judgment, and planning during mealtime (Martin, et al., 1992). In many of these cases, a short period of indirect diagnostic therapy may be warranted to assist the caregiver with carrying out appropriate bolus volumes and feeding rates identified during the videofluorographic examination. When diet modifications (e.g., purees and thickened liquids) or rather laborious feeding methods (e.g., controlled bolus volumes and double swallows) are indicated, a period of calorie and fluid intake measures also should be included as indirect management, because these factors may influence the patient's motivation and potential for sufficient oral intake.

Suggestions for secretion management such as the need for pulmonary toileting by a tracheostomy tube or recommendations regarding the frequency of oral or tracheal suctioning are forms of indirect dysphagia intervention. Involvement of interdisciplinary team members such as the dietitian, nutrition support team, and respiratory therapist also represents a form of indirect management. Other indirect methods include

- structuring the eating environment
- modifying utensils
- specifying the degree of supervision required for safe oral intake (Hotaling, 1990)

DIRECT MANAGEMENT

There are several types of direct management procedures including

- cognitive stimulation
- sensory stimulation
- physiotherapy

- compensatory postures/positioning
- compensatory maneuvers
- assistive devices

The selection of a direct intervention procedure is based on the nature of the swallowing disorder and the patient's level of response. Table 6-1 highlights each of these direct management procedures and indicates those disorders for which they may be appropriate. The reader should also be aware of evolving surgical and medical treatments for selected types of dysphagic impairments that go beyond the scope of this chapter (Aki & Blakely, 1974; Blakely, Garety, & Smith, 1968; Butcher, 1982; Dworkin & Nadal, 1991).

Cognitive Stimulation

The initial goal of treatment is to maximize the awareness and understanding of the swallowing impairment by the patient, physician, nurse, interdisciplinary team members, and caregiver(s). The nature of the swallowing disorder, safety precautions, nutritional requirements, diet modifications, and the rationale for treatment methods are explained. As simple and as obvious as these goals may seem, swallowing clinicians occasionally become so involved in the treatment regime that they do not facilitate active involvement by the patient, family, and involved personnel in the swallowing rehabilitation process. This type of facilitation and education not only eliminates the mystery associated with the swallowing problem but also enhances patient motivation during treatment and carry-over of learned strategies.

It is recommended that the taped videofluorographic examination be reviewed with the patient and family. The role of videofluoroscopy as an important biofeedback tool has been described (Linden, 1989). A patient is more likely to implement the effective pharyngeal clearance strategies if he or she is able to visualize the presence of the pharyngeal residue that occurred during the radiographic examination. Also, direct observation of contrast material entering the laryngeal vestibule will likely promote improved appreciation for the need to use protective airway maneuvers in the case of the noncompliant patient. Depending on the logistics of the health care setting, the inpatient's nurse or outpatient's swallowing clinician should also be encouraged to attend the examination or later review the videotape.

Adjunct diagnostic methods, such as ultrasonography, may be implemented as biofeedback techniques that are visualized by the patient in an attempt to promote lingual bolus control and coordinated tongue movement during the oral stage of swallow (Shawker, Sonies, Hall, & Baum, 1984a; Shawker, Sonies, & Stone, 1984b; Sonies, 1991; Wein, Bockler, & Klajman, 1991). Repeated electromyographic (Bryant, 1991) and manometric studies (Logemann & Kahrilas, 1990; McConnel, 1988) may be conducted over the course of treatment and used to demonstrate increases toward target levels of strength and pressure exerted by the tongue and the pharynx during swallow. Fiberoptic endoscopy allows visualization of laryngeal valving during compensatory breath-hold-

Table 6-1 Differential Dysphagia Diagnosis and Management

Etiology	Clinical Presentation	Radiographic Presentation	Cognitive and Sensory Stimulation	Physiotherapy	Posture/Positioning	Maneuver	Assistive Device
Unilateral or bilateral labial weakness/paralysis with or without impaired bilateral or unilateral labial sensation	Incomplete lip closure Drooling	Incomplete labial seal Escapage of liquid and semisolids Pocketing of foods in anterior oral sulcus	Thickened liquids Intraoral placement to unimpaired side Cold liquids and semisolids	Labial resistive exercises	Head 90°	Lip pursing	Compensatory feeding utensils
Unilateral weakness/paralysis of facial and masticatory musculature	Facial asymmetry Pocketing of foods in oral cavity Labored chewing	Unilateral entrapment of foods in lateral sulcus Inefficient mastication Prolonged bolus preparation	Intraoral placement to unimpaired side Soft solids	Buccal resistive exercises Buccal range of motion exercises	Head tilt to unimpaired side		
Intraoral hyposensitivity	Pooled oral secretions Reduced frequency of saliva swallows Patient reliance on oral suctioning	Diffuse spreading of bolus in oral cavity	Cold liquid/food stimuli Facilitate frequency of dry swallows				
Impaired motor planning and initiation of goal-directed behavior	Slow initiation of oral bolus transport	Delayed initiation of posteriorward bolus movement	Verbal cueing Optimize liquid/food texture Sufficient bolus volumes Cold liquid/food stimuli				
Restricted lingual elevation Restricted lingual lateralization Reduced strength and coordination of lingual motility	Articulatory imprecision Prolonged oral bolus transport Pocketing of foods in oral cavity	Prolonged oral bolus transport Oral residue • tongue dorsum • hard palate • soft palate • floor of mouth • lateral sulci	Intraoral placement to least impaired side Optimize liquid/food texture	Lingual range of motion exercises Lingual resistive exercises Bolus control exercises	Head tilt to unimpaired side	Double swallow	Palatal augmentation prosthesis
Soft palatal weakness/paralysis	Hypernasality Liquids misdirect through nasal cavity	Regurgitation into nasal cavity Oral residue • soft palate • tongue back					Palatal lift prosthesis

continues

Table 6-1 Differential Dysphagia Diagnosis and Management (continued)

Etiology	Clinical Presentation	Radiographic Presentation	Cognitive and Sensory Stimulation	Physiotherapy	Posture/ Positioning	Maneuver	Assistive Device
Incomplete glossopalatal seal (tongue back-velum)	Immediate cough or throat clear	Laryngeal vestibular penetration/aspiration before swallow—premature spillage into pharynx	Controlled bolus volume; Thickened liquids and semisolids	Bolus hold exercises; Lingual resistive exercises (tongue back)		Supraglottic swallow	Palatal augmentation prosthesis
Delayed pharyngeal swallow	Immediate cough or throat clear	Laryngeal vestibular penetration/aspiration before swallow—premature spillage into pharynx; Laryngeal vestibular penetration/aspiration during swallow—pyriform stasis	Cold stimulus; Thickened liquids; Controlled bolus volume; Thermal stimulation	Bolus hold exercises	Chin tuck	Supraglottic swallow	
Incomplete laryngeal elevation and closure • incomplete laryngeal valving • reduced extent and duration of pharyngoesophageal segment opening	Immediate cough or throat clear; Wet vocal quality; Throat clearing after swallows; Multiple effortful swallows per bolus	Incomplete epiglottic descent; Laryngeal vestibular penetration/aspiration during swallow; Laryngeal vestibular penetration/aspiration after swallow—pyriform residue (bilateral)	Controlled bolus volume; Slightly thickened liquids and thinned semisolids	Mendelsohn maneuver; Laryngeal valving exercises		Mendelsohn maneuver; Supraglottic swallow	
Incomplete tongue base retraction	Delayed cough or throat clear; Wet vocal quality	Laryngeal vestibular penetration/aspiration after swallow—vallecular residue	Liquids and semi or soft solids; Controlled bolus volume	Hard swallow; Mendelsohn maneuver	Head/trunk 45–60°	Hard swallow; Double swallow	
Slow return of larynx/ epiglottis	Multiple swallows with solid foods	Vallecular residue	Liquids and soft solids			Double swallow	
Unilateral pharyngeal weakness	Delayed cough or throat clear; Wet vocal quality	Pyriform sinus residue (unilateral) ± pharyngeal diverticula; Residue on pharyngeal wall (unilateral)-penetration/aspiration after swallow	Controlled bolus volume; Liquids, semisolids, and soft solids	Hard swallow	Head/trunk 45–60°; Head rotation toward impaired side; Head tilt toward unimpaired side	Modified supraglottic swallow; Double swallow	
Impaired cricopharyngeal relaxation	Delayed cough or throat clear; Multiple effortful swallows per bolus; Wet vocal quality	Pyriform sinus residue (bilateral) ± pharyngeal diverticula-penetration/ aspiration after swallow	Controlled bolus volume; Liquids and thinned semisolids		Head/trunk 45–60°; Head rotation	Modified supraglottic swallow; Double Swallow	
Pharyngoesophageal segment hypotonicity; Slow esophageal motility	Throat clearing after swallow; Gagging	Regurgitation from esophagus to pyriform sinuses	Liquids, semisolids, and soft solids; Controlled bolus volumes		Head/trunk 45–60°	Double swallow; Modified supraglottic swallow	

ing strategies and may be an effective biofeedback technique when patients are learning laryngeal valving maneuvers (Bastian, 1991; Langmore, Schatz, & Olsen, 1988; Martin et al., 1993). Each or a combination of these strategies serves to promote patient understanding, self-monitoring, and ultimately greater progress toward the acquisition of functional swallowing ability.

A final and obvious form of cognitive stimulation is verbal cueing. The degree of cueing used by the swallowing clinician will depend on the degree of impairment, complexity of the rehabilitation strategy, and the patient's communicative and cognitive status. Postsurgical patients who have become reliant on self-suctioning methods may have "forgotten" how to swallow and warrant step-by-step instructions regarding how to initiate a swallow. Dysphagic patients who have suffered frontal cortical lesions may experience difficulty initiating any goal-directed behavior, including swallowing. Simply saying "Swallow" after placing the stimulus in the oral cavity may not result in the desired response from these types of patients. Often they require cues to close their lips, move their tongue, and "think" swallow.

Sensory Stimulation

Direct swallowing management that uses sensory stimulation is aimed toward heightening the sensitivity of sensory receptive fields that are involved in the facilitation, initiation, efficiency, and safety of deglutition. Sensory stimulation includes

- alterations in food placement within the oral cavity
- modifications in bolus characteristics (i.e., texture, volume, temperature, and taste)
- direct application of sensory treatments to regions of the lips, oral cavity, and oral pharynx

Modifying Food Placement within the Oral Cavity

Dysphagic patients may present with partial or complete sensory loss within the oral cavity related to central or peripheral neurologic insults secondary to stroke, progressive disease, or surgical ablation. The resultant deficits in oral stereognosis negatively influence oral bolus control and safety, the psychological pleasure associated with eating and drinking, and ultimately the patient's nutritional status. In the case of the head and neck cancer patient, this oral sensory deficit may be later confounded by adverse effects of radiotherapy such as xerostomia and soreness. It is the role of the clinician to locate the position in the oral cavity that enhances the patient's ability to feel the location of the bolus to maintain and transport it safely through the oral cavity.

Alterations in intraoral bolus placement can improve swallow efficiency and safety, not only in patients with impaired labial and facial sensation but also in cases of impaired facial and lingual muscle strength. During normal deglutition, food is masticated by alternating the bolus from the surfaces of the molars to the tongue and then recollected to form a cohesive bolus before oral transport (Logemann, 1983). Intact facial muscle tone and interdental contact result in the establishment of lateral walls that maintain the bolus in an optimal position in the oral chamber during mastication. After bolus preparation, the material is held in the oral cavity by elevated tongue margins that approximate the palate anteriorly, laterally, and posteriorly. If the integrity of the facial or lingual muscles is disturbed, the bolus spreads throughout the oral cavity and may be emitted through the lips or fall prematurely over the back of the tongue and into the pharynx. In such cases of reduced oral control, the region of the oral cavity that facilitates optimum bolus hold and transport must be identified and used during feedings. Also, increasing the viscosity of the food/liquid stimuli in these cases of oral sensory or motor dysfunction will reduce the tendency for the material to escape from the oral cavity.

Modifying Bolus Characteristics

The influences of bolus characteristics on the normal physiology of swallow have been recognized since the time of the first cineradiographic observations (Ardran & Kemp, 1952, 1967; Ramsey, Watson, Gramiak, & Weinberg, 1955). Refined analysis of videofluorographic swallowing studies using measured volumes of barium revealed that the duration of hyolaryngeal excursion, laryngeal vestibular closure, and the extent and duration of pharyngoesophageal sphincter (PES) opening are modulated with graduated bolus volumes and alternate bolus textures in normal adult subjects (Dantes et al., 1990; Jacob, Kahrilas, Logemann, Shah, & Ha, 1989; Lof & Robbins, 1990; Logemann et al., 1992; Tracy et al., 1989; Veis, Logemann, & Kahrilas, 1989).

Clinical observations support these findings that bolus characteristics have appreciable effect on the onset and duration of swallowing events and warrant careful scrutiny during the videofluoroscopic evaluation. Gradations of bolus volume and texture should be implemented during the examination to determine the optimum bolus characteristics used in swallowing therapy. The clinician must be careful to recognize that there are no steadfast rules regarding which food or liquid textures are optimal for different categories of patients. Well-controlled studies that have applied different food or liquid textures in specific groups of dysphagic patient populations and studied their effects on the physiology of swallowing have not been performed. Therefore, the treatment suggestions listed in Table 6-1 should serve only as general guidelines, and their effectiveness must be validated during the videofluoroscopic evaluation for each individual patient.

Modifying Bolus Texture

Thick liquids are often tolerated more safely than thin liquids in patients with delayed initiation of the pharyngeal swallow because viscous substances fall less rapidly than diluted liquids. A thick liquid is less likely to fall forward into the laryngeal inlet during the delay before pharyngeal swallow initiation as compared with the free-fall behavior of thin liquids (Fig. 6-1). Also, viscous materials may result in increased tongue movement with enhanced displacement of mechanoreceptors when compared with thin liquid consistencies and facilitate more timely initiation of the pharyngeal swallow. A patient presenting with incomplete laryngeal elevation and closure may also benefit from a viscous liquid during swallow. A thick liquid is less likely than a thin liquid to penetrate the incompletely sealed larynx (Fig. 6-2).

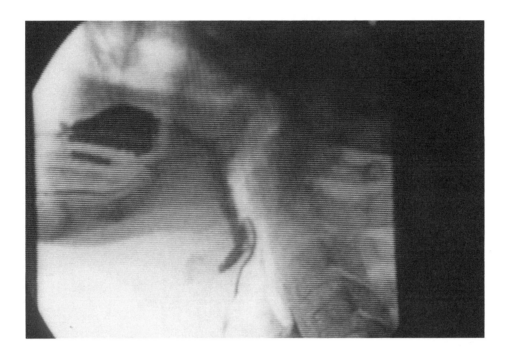

A

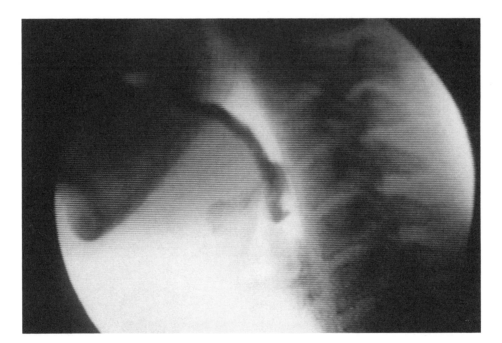

B

Fig. 6-1 Delayed Initiation of Pharyngeal Swallow. **(A)** A Thin Liquid Bolus Falls Rapidly into Pharynx and Misdirects to Laryngeal Vestibule. **(B)** Laryngeal Penetration Is Prevented as Viscous Liquid Remains in Pharyngeal Recesses.

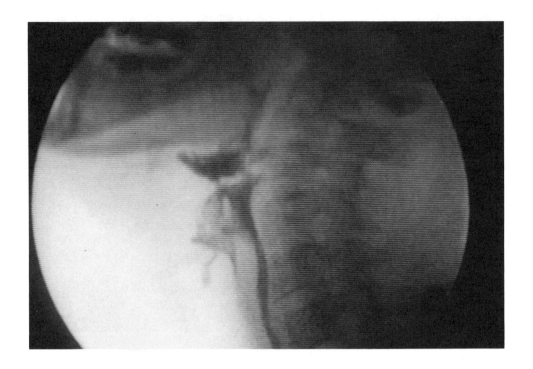

A

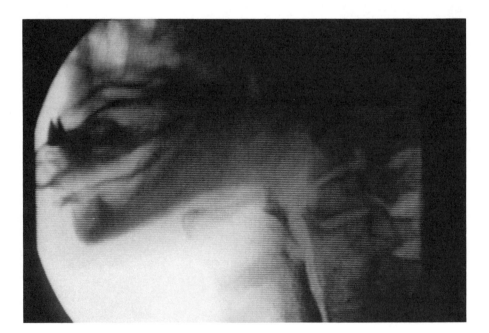

B

Fig. 6-2   Reduction in Laryngeal Elevation and Closure. **(A)** Large Volume Thin Liquid Bolus Is Likely to Penetrate Laryngeal Vestibule during Swallow. **(B)** Laryngeal Penetration Is Prevented with a Controlled (2- to 5-mL) Thickened Liquid Bolus.

Despite the advantages of thickened liquid in the management of dysphagic patients, the clinician is reminded that impaired swallow components rarely occur in isolation but rather in combination with overlapping impairments of the oral cavity, pharynx, larynx, and esophagus. Viscous materials will not improve the safety of swallow if the delayed pharyngeal swallow is combined with a significant inability to clear the pharynx of thick materials. Further, even though the introduction of liquid thickening agents have come to be an invaluable means of dysphagia management, careful attention must be given to their effect on the adequacy of a patient's hydration. The physiologic work associated with swallowing thickened liquid increases, and the satiation of thirst is usually reported as diminished. Therefore, careful planning must be coordinated between physician, nurse, and clinical nutritionist to ensure that the patient's hydration needs are met.

Health care professionals occasionally overgeneralize the use of thickened liquids as an aspiration remedy for all dysphagic patients regardless of the nature of impairment and unfortunately fail to refer the patients for appropriate diagnostic evaluations. The swallowing clinician has the responsibility to educate the health care team as to the advantages and disadvantages of thickened liquids and to the necessity for the radiographic evaluation in delineating the optimum bolus characteristics. Another example of an overgeneralization is that all stroke patients with dysphagia be administered pureed foods. Although this recommendation may be valid in the case of inefficient mastication and slow lingual motility, there are occasions when soft or solid foods seem to provide the necessary oral sensory stimulation for the initiation of productive mastication and lingual motility. Further, the motivation for oral intake may be negatively altered after several weeks or months of pureed meals. This problem taxes the creativity of the swallowing clinician, nutritionist, and meal planner.

Modifying Bolus Volume

The individuality of effective bolus characteristics for swallow facilitation is exemplified not only in the texture of the bolus but also in the bolus volume. Recommended liquid volumes during the radiographic swallow study include 2 ml (i.e., approximately $^1/_2$ teaspoon), 5 ml (1 teaspoon), 10 ml (small sip), and 20 ml (average bolus in normal adults). (Adnerhill, Ekberg, & Groher, 1989). The determination of each increase should be dependent on the patient's ability to manage the preceding smaller volume safely. The rationale for providing a patient with small volume boluses is to prevent or minimize the degree of aspiration that may occur. If a patient demonstrates the tendency toward aspiration during a pharyngeal swallow delay, a smaller bolus will not enter the pharynx as rapidly as a larger volume and may fill the valleculae until airway closure is initiated during the swallow (Fig. 6-3). If the bolus progresses further to the pyriform sinuses during the delay, a small amount of liquid or food in the pyriform pocket will less likely flow into the laryngeal inlet before the pharyngeal swallow initiation or later during elevation of the larynx. It has also been shown that the duration of swallow apnea positively correlates with the duration of laryngeal elevation and closure (Martin, 1991). This may place a patient with pulmonary dysfunction at a swallow safety disadvantage if he or she is unable to maintain the prolonged laryngeal closure that is associated with large volume swallows.

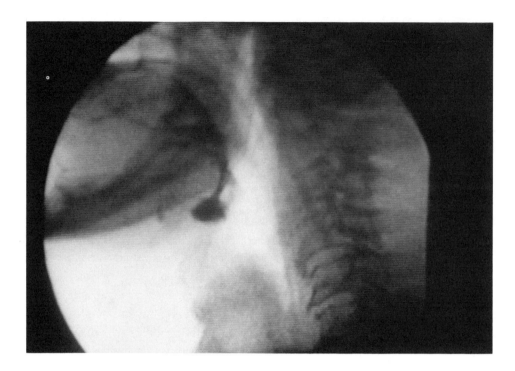

Fig. 6-3 Delayed Pharyngeal Swallow. Small Bolus Is Retained in the Valleculae by Upright Epiglottis

In contrast, there have been cases observed during videofluoroscopy that require a substantial bolus volume for a patient to initiate oral bolus transport. Perhaps additional sensory receptive fields must be stimulated in patients who experience difficulty initiating this volitional behavior. Further, because increased bolus volumes increase the extent and duration of laryngeal elevation, laryngeal closure, and pharyngoesophageal segment opening, some dysphagic patients without significant respiratory impairment may benefit from these modulating bolus characteristics (Jacob et al., 1989; Lof & Robbins, 1990; Tracy et al., 1989; Veis et al., 1989). Caution must be taken to test these hypotheses during the radiographic evaluation.

Modifying Bolus Temperature and Taste

The ideal bolus temperature for swallow facilitation also appears to be quite variable from patient to patient. In patients with blunted oral sensation or poor initiation of oral bolus transport, a cold stimulus seems to facilitate more rapid posteriorward tongue movement and pharyngeal swallow elicitation. However, there are some dysphagic patients with chronic respiratory problems who perceive cold as a noxious stimulus and swallow more precipitously and efficiently with a tepid or warm bolus.

The gustatory characteristics of the bolus also tend to be quite variable, depending on the premorbid preferences of the patient and on alterations in taste after the neurologic, surgical, or medical insult. Given the individuality of these stimulus characteristics as they relate to swallow facilitation, the clinician should include an inventory of taste and temperature preferences as part of the diagnostic and therapy regime.

Effects of Pain

Final consideration in this discussion of sensory attributes of swallow should be given to the issue of pain (i.e., odynophagia), or other swallow-related discomfort. The influence of pain on normal swallow dynamics has not been studied and is difficult to measure because most patients with pain have dysphagia-related diseases or conditions that precipitate the pain. Although it seems increasingly difficult for an otherwise healthy individual to swallow when experiencing a sore throat, the potential alterations in swallow mechanics is uncertain. The author has observed cases wherein a patient presents with an infection or irritation to the mucosal linings of the mouth and throat. Based on the patient's complaints of swallowing difficulty, they were seen for videofluoroscopic evaluation. Significant deviations from normal swallow mechanics were occasionally observed in these patients. It is unknown to what degree these changes were caused by the pain or to patient compensation attempts to minimize the pain associated with swallow. Nonetheless, particularly in patients undergoing treatments for head and neck cancers or prolonged naso-oral and tracheal intubation, the contribution of pain and discomfort to their dysphagia should not be trivialized. When treating these patients, it may be effective to request that pain medication be administered before their swallowing therapy sessions to exclude this intervening variable. However, some topical anesthetics applied to the oral cavity and pharynx may be contraindicated during and around the time of therapy because of their probable tendency to further diminish sensory input to swallow.

Thermal Stimulation

The treatment "thermal stimulation" is described as the application of light pressure to the anterior fauces in a series of taps or strokes using a cold 00 laryngeal mirror and is recommended for use with patients who present with delayed initiation of the pharyngeal swallow (Logemann, 1983). This sensory treatment was developed from the findings of early swallow stimulation studies and clinical practice (Lazzara, Lazarus, & Logemann, 1986; Mansson & Sandberg, 1975; Pommerenke, 1928). It is based on the hypothesis that mechanical and thermal sensory receptors in the anterior oropharynx are the most reflexogenic for swallow elicitation and, when mechanically stimulated with a blunt cold object, will heighten the sensitivity and timing of the pharyngeal swallow (Lazzara et al., 1986). One investigative report described improvement in the timing and initiation of swallow in dysphagic individuals immediately after the treatment was applied (Lazzara et al., 1986). A more recent study, however, did not find substantial differences in patient swallow recovery after undergoing routine application of the technique compared with patients who did not receive this treatment (Rosenbeck, Robbins, Fishback, & Levine, 1991).

Although clinical experience indicates that the technique has treatment use with select dysphagic patients, there is insufficient data regarding its role or effectiveness in swallow facilitation. The efficacy of its use is further complicated by the fact that the neural initiation of swallow in adult humans is not completely understood. However, the author has found the method to be useful in patients with delayed pharyngeal swallows but only when combined with other input modalities including cognitive stimulation and the presence of a bolus. The most desirable outcomes have been achieved when the stimulation is applied and followed by the introduction of a 1-mL water bolus into the floor of the patient's oral cavity with a pipette. The use of a 1-mL bolus after thermal stimulation approximates a normal saliva swallow and is unlikely to result in patient complication. A neutral, sterile substance such as saline could also be administered in lieu of water. The patient is then cued to move their tongue and swallow. If an oral stimulus or tongue movement is not included with the thermal stimulation, experience has shown that a swallow typically does not ensue. This is not surprising based on the clinical observations that swallow is a response to multiple sensory stimuli and that patients respond optimally to the application of multiple sensory stimulation (i.e., resence of a bolus, tongue movement). The integrated verbal cueing encourages the patient to "think swa low" and gives a goal to achieve after application of the treatment. There will be cases in which the patient will be unable to respond to this type of verbal cueing, and the effectiveness of the treatment is significantly diminished. Another complicating factor concerning thermal stimulation is whether the neural pathway for swallowing is susceptible to hyperpolarization (i.e., inhibited secondary to overstimulation) (Kandel, 1985). The clinician should take steps to avoid the possibility of hyperpolarization. Therefore, thermal stimulation should probably be performed for short periods and several times throughout the day.

The significance of an oral stimulus was elucidated in a recent pilot investigation (Martin et al., 1992). At rest, young healthy subjects were found to swallow about one time per minute in either the supine or sitting position. However, when a lozenge was inserted into the oral cavity, the frequency of swallow increased threefold. The cause of increased swallow frequency cannot be determined from this work but probably represents a combination of inputs such as

- pressure applied to the tongue
- facilitory tongue movement during sucking
- increased salivary production (Sonies, Ship, & Baum, 1989)

Although we are not proposing the introduction of oral stimuli in all patients, this simple technique may be a viable means of swallow facilitation when controlled by the clinician in appropriate patient groups.

Physiotherapy

Physiotherapeutic exercises are applied to the striated muscles of the impaired oral cavity, pharynx, larynx, and cervical esophagus much in the same way as they are applied to impaired musculature of the extremities. The goal of these exercises is to strengthen the motor unit and to improve the range, speed, and coordination of movement.

Increased range of movement could be measured with scales or by plotting the distances of structural movement over time during swallow (Caruso, Stanhope, & McGuire, 1989; Dengel, Robbins, & Rosenbeck, 1991; Logemann, Kahrilas, Begelman, Dodds, & Pauloski, 1989a). Increased strength or amplitude of contraction could be measured with electromyography of specific muscles and groups of muscles or may be inferred through pressure readings obtained from manometric studies (Bryant, 1991; Logemann & Kahrilas, 1990; Perlman et al., 1989). To date, however, these techniques are not widespread and have not been tested on large numbers of normal or dysphagic patients. Therefore, until we progress further in our studies of treatment effectiveness, we rely on the implementation of those physiotherapeutic techniques that appear to have been effective throughout our clinical practices with dysphagic patients.

Range

The term *range* as it appears in the contexts of this chapter refers to an individual's ability to effect a given distance or extent of muscle movement. Treatment techniques are aimed toward increased displacement of a structure or muscle group. However, passive range of motion activities do not show clinical use for patients with oropharyngeal swallowing impairments. Rather, the patient must have the cognitive ability to follow at least one-step instructions and be able to imitate isolated orofacial movements.

Patients with neurologic injuries to the central or peripheral nervous system may present with limitations in the range of oral, facial, pharyngeal, and laryngeal movement. Individuals with head and neck cancers often suffer from isolated restrictions in range of labial or lingual movements, secondary to surgical removal of muscles, bone, and connective tissues. Depending on the locus of the applied oncologic treatments, there may also be restriction of mouth opening caused by disruption in attachments of the muscles of the mandible. Further, postoperative or primary radiation treatment may result in tissue changes, such as fibrosis, that cause rigidity in different muscles and joints. The nature of the surgical closure may result in limited range of labial and lingual motion necessary for oral bolus control and transport. Clinical attempts to facilitate increased range of movement in these patient populations can be effective in the recovery of the functional swallow.

Increasing Range of Mandibular Movements

Mastication is a complex physiologic activity that requires mandibular lateralization and elevation (Palmer, Rudin, Lara, & Crompton, 1992). Lateral mandibular movement can be promoted by asking the patient to imitate alternating left to right jaw extensions. The lateral rotary-like jaw movement observed during mastication can also be practiced by the patient as he or she attempts to chew a soft piece of chewing gum tied to a string that is held by the clinician. When the clinician is concerned about the patient's ability to maintain any bolus within the oral cavity, the patient could perform light chewing strokes against the tip of a soft-sponged toothette held firmly by the clinician. In patients who demonstrate restricted range of mouth opening (i.e., mandibular depression), a bite block made of soft material of different widths may be applied interdentally between the central incisors to facilitate a gradual increase in the distance between the upper and lower teeth. Using a mirror, the patient later attempts to match the opening width without the use of the bite block device. In the case of the patient with an exaggerated bite response, systematic desensitization techniques should be used (Brown, Nordloh, & Donowitz, 1992). Attempts to pry the mouth open are not the recommended method of management. Rather, the jaw may be pushed closed and held firmly for a few seconds. When the pressure is released, jaw relaxation should result (Umphred & McCormack, 1985).

Another frequently occurring problem is difficulty achieving mouth closure (i.e., mandibular elevation). Oral cancer patients may be unable to feel the position of the oral structures because of temporarily diminished orofacial sensation. This may result in a lowered mandible and profuse drooling between the parted lips. In contrast, an open mouth posture may result also in excessive xerostomia and accumulation of dry oral mucus. Particular attention to oral care by the nursing staff is warranted in this patient group, and the swallowing clinician is often the first to recognize inadequate oral hygiene. Patients who breathe through their mouth, such as those with indwelling nasogastric (NG) tubes or chronic pulmonary problems often demonstrate these patterns and may require instruction to elevate the mandible to improve intraoral hydration and facilitation of a functional swallow. In these patients, the problem is typically not with restricted range of mandibular movement but with lack of awareness and diminished sensory stimulation. Therefore, any activity that promotes improved patient awareness and tongue movement should facilitate mandibular elevation with mouth closure, salivation, and swallow.

Any exercise that is directed toward increasing the range of mandibular elevation will result in improved approximation of the upper and lower lips. Patients with limitations in range can be instructed to imitate lateral and medial labial movements to prevent stiffening and enhance mobility of the lips for speech, swallowing, and physical appearance. On each trial, the patient should be instructed to maintain the targeted lip posture for a few seconds before return to the rest position.

Increasing Range of Lingual Movements

Head and neck cancer patients who have undergone surgeries to the oral cavity including the tongue and/or floor of mouth may exhibit significant isolated problems involving restricted range of tongue lateralization, elevation, and posterior retraction. Tongue lateralization can be facilitated in this population by having the patient imitate alternating lateral movements of the tongue tip while viewing his or her performance in front of a mirror. A main objective of the exercise is for the patient to sustain the isolated posture. Approximation of the tongue tip toward the alveolus should also be imitated to enhance lingual elevation. During both of these activities, the clinician should manually stabilize the jaw to maximize the work of the tongue musculature and connective tissue. The practical objective of tongue range of motion exercises is improved tongue lateralization and elevation that will result in efficient mastication and oral bolus control. Therefore, the clinician should gradually incorporate an oral stimulus into the exercises. The patient should learn to cup or seal a controlled bolus to the hard palate and to simulate chewing through manipulation of a bolus from the tongue to the margins of the lateral teeth. The nature of the bolus will be dependent on the severity of the impairment and on the cognitive status of the patient. Examples of stimuli include a moistened, soft-sponged toothette, flavored suckers, or rolled pieces of flavored gauze held at one end by the clinician. Sticky foods such as peanut butter or frosting may be placed on the hard palate, and the patient is asked to scrape the material from the palate with the tongue. Care must be taken for the patient to expectorate the retrieved material when indicated.

Increases in range of posterior tongue elevation may be facilitated by manually depressing the back of the tongue with a tongue blade and asking the patient to displace the tongue upward against the blade. The resistance offered by the tongue blade will also promote strengthening of muscles in the body of the tongue.

It is also important to consider the base of the tongue. After entry of the bolus into the pharynx, the tongue base thrusts posteriorly to approximate the pharyngeal walls and drives the material through the pharyngeal cavity. When range of tongue base movement is restricted, there will be considerable residue in the pharynx, primarily in the valleculae and on the posterior pharyngeal wall, which increases the threat of residue aspiration (Perlman, Grayhack, & Booth, 1992). An exercise that has been observed to be effective in increasing the range of tongue base retraction is asking the patient to "swallow hard." Using this technique, patients can learn to effect a greater posteriorward excursion, and there appears to be an accompanying increase in strength of tongue movement and degree of laryngeal closure and pharyngeal contraction.

Strengthening

Dysphagic patients frequently present with overlapping weakness of musculature of the oral cavity, pharynx, and larynx. Striated muscles of the aerodigestive tract contract to perform mechanical work, and resistance is used to facilitate muscle contraction (Umphred & McCormack, 1985). Resistive exercises may be applied to the muscles of the lips and tongue.

Resistive labial exercises are directed toward improved integrity of the lip seal to maintain foods and liquids in the oral cavity. Improved labial strength can be facilitated by asking the patient to purse the lips tightly to each other for approximately 5 seconds, followed by a slow release. An additional activity includes pursing the lips against an intervening tongue blade while the clinician attempts to pull the blade from the lips. Increased lip strength is also facilitated when a patient attempts to maintain a moist soft-sponged toothette or swab in the oral cavity with pursed lips while the clinician attempts to withdraw this stimulus.

Similar resistive exercises can be used to promote improved strength of lingual musculature. A patient's application of tongue pressure in lateral and upward directions against a tongue blade facilitates strengthening of the extrinsic muscles of the tongue during the exercise. Increased intrinsic muscle strength required for elevation of the anterior, lateral, and posterior margins can be chieved by having the dysphagic patient cup a stimulus to the hard palate while the clinician attempts its removal. The oral stimuli that may be chosen by the clinician would be similar to those described in the previous section and must be selected based on the nature of the impairment. When a patient is able to tolerate controlled boluses of thick liquids and semisolids safely, these materials may be used during the progressive strengthening exercise program. In these cases, the patient is asked to hold the bolus tightly in the oral cavity by contracting intrinsic and extrinsic lingual musculature and to prevent escape of the bolus to the oral sulci, floor of mouth, and pharynx. This type of oral control also requires a downward and forwardly displaced tonic soft palate that seals to the back of tongue and further prevents premature spillage into the pharynx. Therefore, this activity may also facilitate improved strength of the palatoglossus muscle.

Besides the downward and forward action, elevation and retraction of the soft palate (i.e., contraction of the levator veli palatini muscle) are also required during swallow to effect velopharyngeal valving and prevent misdirection of foods or liquids into the nasal cavity. However, it is difficult to apply resistive therapeutic activities that promote increased strength of the levator muscle, and a flaccid or surgically altered soft palate is typically managed by fitting the patient with an obturating palatal augmentation prosthesis (Logemann, Kahrilas, Hurst, Davis, & Krugler, 1989b).

Compensatory Postures and Positions

Ideally, compensatory postures should serve as temporary methods during the recovery of an impaired aerodigestive tract to facilitate the efficiency and safety of bolus passage through the oral cavity, pharynx, and esophagus. However, there are cases of severe swallowing impairment that require the permanent employment of these alternate postures. Four postures have been described (Logemann, 1983):

- chin down
- head back
- head tilt
- head rotation

The implementation of the postures must be based on the nature of the patient's swallowing deficits and intact swallowing components, and their effectiveness should be objectively tested during the videofluoroscopic examination.

The chin-down posture serves as an effective airway protective position in appropriate patients who present with delayed initiation of the pharyngeal swallow (Table 6-1). When the chin is tucked to the chest, the tongue is drawn forward and the vallecular space is widened (Logemann, 1983). The widened vallecular space results in a wider weigh station for hesitated material during the swallow delay, thereby preventing or minimizing premature entry of the bolus into the pharynx and open larynx. The open larynx, which does not begin its valving or closure until the pharyngeal swallow is initiated, is also drawn forward and is somewhat channeled under the tongue base as a result of the tucked chin posture. The open laryngeal vestibule is therefore less vulnerable to penetration because it receives additional protection from the tongue.

The chin-down posture has often been inappropriately applied to all types of swallowing impairment that result in laryngeal penetration and/or aspiration. It should be recognized that the head tuck is not a panacea for all swallowing problems and may even promote aspiration in some cases. If the delayed initiation of the pharyngeal swallow is confounded by a reduction in laryngeal elevation and closure, the chin-down posture may facilitate forward misdirection of liquid or food into the airway during the swallow. Also, if the posture is not combined with bolus volume control, the large thin liquid bolus will fill the valleculae, overflow into the pharynx, and misdirect to the laryngeal inlet. Furthermore, if the delay is so significant that the pharyngeal swallow does not trigger until materials reach the pyriform sinuses, then the hesitated material in the pyriforms will likely divert anteriorly into the airway during laryngeal elevation. The efficiency of the maneuver must also be considered. A chin-down posture will result in inefficient oral bolus containment, control, and transport if there is sensorimotor impairment of the lips and tongue.

A less frequently used posture is the head-back position. The use of this approach is highlighted in the patient with poor lingual motility for oral bolus transport, but who otherwise exhibits good airway closure and pharyngeal clearance. This method may be especially effective in the head and neck cancer patient after oral resections; however, many patients complain that it is difficult for them to swallow with backward flexion of the head and neck. There are also obvious dangers of using this technique with cognitively impaired patients who exhibit incomplete laryngeal closure.

Head-tilt and head-rotation postures may be implemented with patients suffering from unilateral impairment of the pharynx and cervical esophageal swallowing problems (Logemann, 1983). The head-tilt posture involves the patient tipping the head to the unimpaired or less impaired side to provide more complete pharyngeal clearance. Conversely, the head-rotation posture requires that the patient turn the head toward the side of impairment. The aim of the posture is to prevent bolus transport through the weaker side, thereby preventing or decreasing excess pharyngeal residue after the swallow (Logemann, 1983). It has been further shown that this posture facilitates passage of the bolus into the cervical esophagus, reducing pharyngeal-esophageal sphincter pressure (Logemann, Kahrilas, Kobara, and Vakil, 1989c).

Alterations in body position shown to be effective on the radiographic swallowing evaluations may also be used to facilitate a safe and efficient swallow during oral feedings. Positioning the head and trunk upright to 45 degrees has been shown to be clinically effective in managing aspiration in select dysphagic patients. The use of this position may seem contraindicated because most individuals typically eat when the head and trunk are positioned upright at 90 degrees. However, hospitalized patients often drink and eat in their beds when the head and trunk are upright only 60 to 70 degrees. Therefore, performing a radiographic study at 90 degrees may give an inaccurate profile of their swallowing abilities at the bedside.

When a patient presents with a moderate degree of vallecular or pyriform sinus residue, a 90 degree head–trunk position will most likely facilitate the forward misdirection of the residue resulting from gravitational effects on the bolus (Fig. 6-4). Therefore, feeding the patient in the 45 degree head–trunk position may be beneficial in the following circumstances:

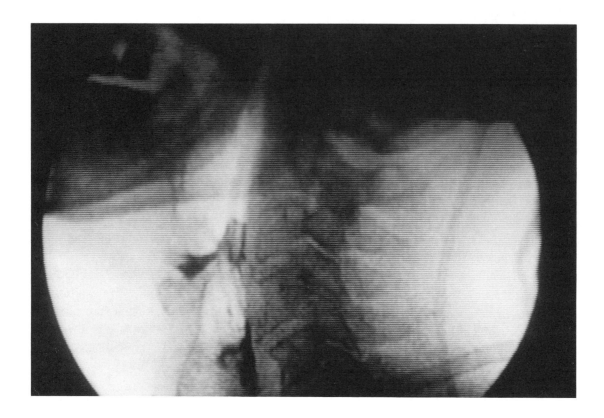

Fig. 6-4 Incomplete Pharyngeal Clearance. The 90 Degree Head–Trunk Position Results in Forward Spill of Residue from the Pharyngeal Valleculae and Pyriform Sinuses

- when there is a rather steady amount of pharyngeal residue after swallow and the patient does not have the cognitive ability to follow each wet swallow with a dry swallow
- when the prognosis for significant return of neuromuscular function required for safe swallowing is poor and the patient/caregivers express a strong desire for some oral intake

The 45 degree angle results in drainage of the residue from the valleculae down the posterior wall and into the pyriform sinuses. A reflexive swallow usually follows, and laryngeal penetration and aspiration may be prevented.

This type of feeding is typically only supplemental to alternative methods of feeding such as NG and gastric tubes or hyperalimentation. Bolus volumes must be kept to a minimum (2 to 5mL), and appropriate texture modifications are required and specified during the videofluoroscopic examination. Further, the clinician must consider the integrity of esophageal motility, clearance, and lower esophageal sphincter function. In patients with significant vagal impairment, especially in the elderly with premorbidly slow esophageal motility, a functional impairment of esophageal peristalsis and clearance may be observed (Fig. 6-5). The compensatory 45 degree head–trunk position usually prevents or minimizes the forward misdirection of regurgitated material from the esophagus into the airway.

Examination of Table 6-1 shows that rarely are compensatory postures or positions used in isolation. Rather, controlled bolus volumes, modified bolus textures, slow feeding rates, and cognitive stimulation are usually combined, depending on the clinical and swallowing problem profile of the dysphagic patient. The use of airway protective swallowing maneuvers are frequently used in conjunction with these compensatory strategies.

Compensatory Maneuvers

Advances in frame-by-frame and biomechanical analysis of swallowing have resulted in an improved understanding of the effects of rehabilitative maneuvers on swallowing physiology (Dengel, et al., 1991; Logemann 1986; Logemann, et al., 1989a). The available compensatory maneuvers vary in their complexity and are useful only with patients who can adequately understand the rationale for the maneuver, follow two- to three-step instructions, and retain instructions over time. Unfortunately, the cognitive skills required for implementation of these maneuvers often precludes their use with many dysphagic patients who present with a high incidence of communication and cognitive impairments (Martin and Corlew, 1990).

Four compensatory swallowing maneuvers will be described that have been shown to improve airway protection and the efficiency of bolus passage through the aerodigestive tract:

- double swallow
- hard swallow
- supraglottic swallow
- Mendelsohn maneuver

Double Swallow

The double swallow is a simple, yet effective compensatory maneuver that involves directing the patient to swallow two or three times per bolus (e.g., after wet swallows with subsequent dry swallows). The number of repetitive dry swallows will vary with the size of the bolus, bolus texture, and severity of impairment. This maneuver may be used with patients who demonstrate incomplete pharyngeal clearance during the initial swallow for a variety of reasons that may include decreased tongue base retraction, reduced laryngeal elevation with accompanying reductions in the extent and duration of pharyngo-esophageal segment opening, and weak contraction of the pharyngeal musculature. The second swallow is also beneficial for patients who present with oral residue related to slow and inefficient lingual motility. Like all the maneuvers that will be described in this text, the double swallow not only serves to improve oropharyngeal clearance but also serves as a physiotherapeutic exercise that probably facilitates improved strength of muscle contraction (Perlman et al., 1989).

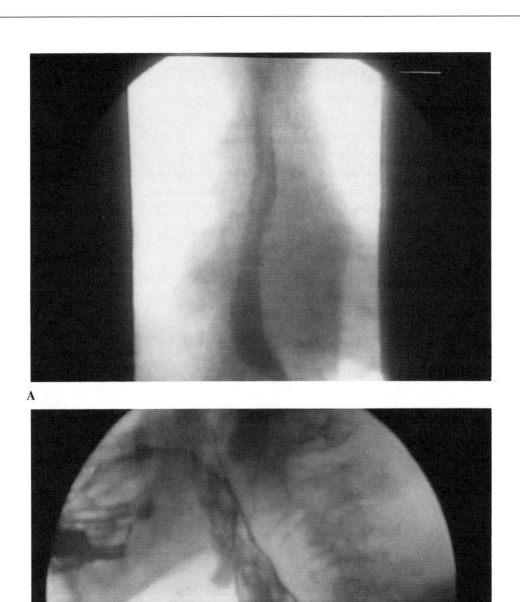

A

B

Fig. 6-5. (A) Slow Esophageal Clearance Resulting from Impaired Peristalsis with Tertiary Contractions; (B) Spontaneous Esophagopharyngeal Regurgitation and Laryngeal Penetration

Hard Swallow

The hard swallow maneuver is used with patients who present with incomplete pharyngeal clearance resulting from incomplete tongue base retraction. When the tongue base does not meet the posterior and lateral pharyngeal walls after entry of the bolus tail into the pharynx, there is inadequate pressure applied to the bolus from above (McConnel, Mendelsohn, & Logemann, 1987). The radiographic symptom is typically excess residue primarily in the vallecula. In these cases, the patient is instructed to swallow hard or with effort and attempt to feel the backward motion of the tongue. The act of swallow has been described as the optimal swallow practice (Linden-Castelli, 1991; Perlman et al., 1989). Therefore, the hard swallow may also be used as a physiotherapeutic exercise. Before beginning oral intake, a hard dry or 1-mL water swallow by severely involved dysphagic patients may facilitate improved strength of tongue base retraction and pharyngeal wall contraction.

Supraglottic Swallow Maneuver

The supraglottic swallow maneuver involves exertion of voluntary control over otherwise involuntary swallow events (Logemann, 1983). The possibility of voluntary airway closure was recognized early when it was found that patients with epiglottic excision learned to close their larynx before swallowing to prevent laryngeal vestibular penetration (Ardran and Kemp, 1952) (Fig. 6-6). These early observations of voluntary laryngeal protection are often found to be useful in the clinical management of select dysphagic patients. Like the other compensatory strategies, the maneuver should be applied to only those patients with swallowing anomalies that have been shown to benefit from such a maneuver during videofluoroscopy (Martin et al., 1993).

The supraglottic swallow involves the following steps:

1. Take and hold a breath.
2. Place food or liquid in the mouth.
3. Swallow (once or twice, depending on the efficiency of pharyngeal clearance).
4. Clear your throat.
5. Swallow again.

The patient is instructed not to re-establish breathing at any point during the sequence to prevent inhalation of pharyngeal stasis (i.e., hesitated food/liquid) or residue (i.e., leftover material after the swallow). The clinician must be careful to instruct the patient to clear the throat "out" rather than to cough, because many patients will attempt to inhale before a coughing maneuver.

The supraglottic swallow is effective in patients who present with

- delayed initiation of pharyngeal swallow
- incomplete supraglottic valving
- incomplete pharyngeal clearance

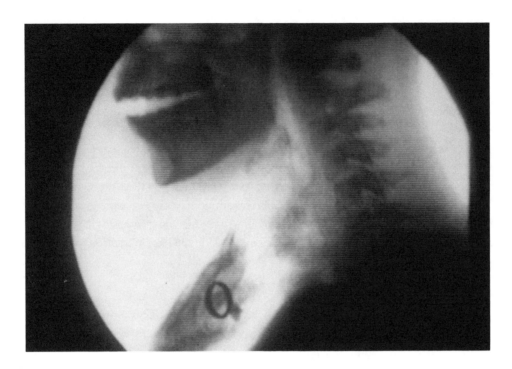

Fig. 6-6 Supraglottic Swallow Characterized by Volitional Closure of Laryngeal Valves Before Pharyngeal Swallow Initiation

The primary goal of the maneuver is to facilitate airway closure before and during the swallow and to clear potential residue, primarily from the laryngeal vestibule and pyriform sinuses. However, a recent study has shown that a breath-hold with fixation of the chest does not ensure glottic closure in normal patients and is probably less likely in patients with significant muscle weakness and poor endurance (Martin et al., 1992). It was found that when patients were instructed to hold their breath hard with effort or to bear down, the degree of laryngeal valving significantly increased (Fig. 6-7). The patient's ability to achieve this type of valving should be confirmed with videofluoroscopy and preferably fiberoptic videonasoendoscopy. The fiberoptic approach provides the clinician with a direct view of laryngeal valving capability and may also serve as an effective biofeedback tool in patient training. However, the patient's ability to maintain laryngeal valving during the swallow is best confirmed by prevention of laryngeal penetration during the swallow as viewed on video-nasendoscopy.

The supraglottic swallow maneuver may be modified for patients who present with incomplete pharyngeal clearance but with good laryngeal closure. In these patients, a breath-hold is not necessary. Rather, they are instructed to double swallow to promote increased clearance, clear their throat to prevent potential entry of pharyngeal residue from entering the laryngeal vestibule, and to swallow a third time.

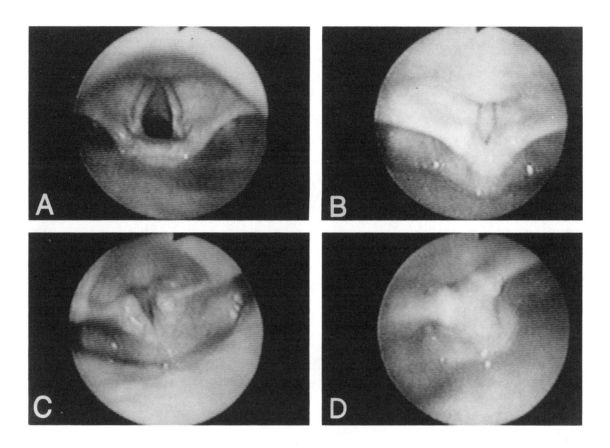

Figure 6-7 Degrees of Laryngeal Valving that Increase as the Subject Exerts Greater Effort: **(A)** Absent Laryngeal Valving; **(B)** Arytenoid Approximation and True Vocal Fold Closure; **(C)** False Vocal Fold Approximation and Anterior Tilt of Arytenoids; **(D)** Arytenoid to Epiglottic Base Contact
Source: Reprinted with permission from *Dysphagia* (1993; 8 [1]: 11–20), Copyright © 1993, Springer-Verlag

A final application of a modified supraglottic maneuver, usually accompanied by the 45–60-degree head–trunk position, is with the patient who exhibits slow transit of material through the thoracic esophagus and occasional regurgitation of the hesitated material into the pyriform sinuses (see Fig. 6-5). If the degree of pharyngeal re-entry is only a trace amount, the throat clear followed by a dry swallow may prevent chronic trace laryngeal penetration or aspiration.

Mendelsohn Maneuver

The Mendelsohn maneuver is effective in patients with incomplete opening or premature closing of the PES. It has been observed that if a patient voluntarily maintains the hyolaryngeal complex in its elevated and anteriorly displaced position during the height of swallow, the PES increased the duration of its opening, and the duration of laryngeal closure and tongue base retraction also increased (Kahrilas, Logemann, Krugler, & Flanagan, 1991; Logemann & Kahrilas, 1990; McConnel, Cerenko, & Mendelsohn, 1988). Patients can be trained to hold the larynx in its involuntarily initiated, elevated position, which facilitates increased extent and duration of PES opening and more complete pharyngeal clearance (Fig. 6-8). A modified supraglottic swallow may be combined with this strategy to prevent trace laryngeal vestibular penetration of pyriform residue that may not have cleared during the maneuver.

The Mendelsohn maneuver has also been observed to be effective as a physiotherapeutic exercise in nonorally fed patients. During dry or 1-mL water swallows, patients are instructed to hold the larynx in the elevated position for 3 to 5 seconds. The exercise is directed toward improving the strength and range of hyolaryngeal elevation and tongue base retraction with patients shown to have deficits in these areas on videofluoroscopy.

The use of compensatory postures and maneuvers can be very effective methods in the clinical management of swallow efficiency and safety. However, the cognitive and "whole body" systems

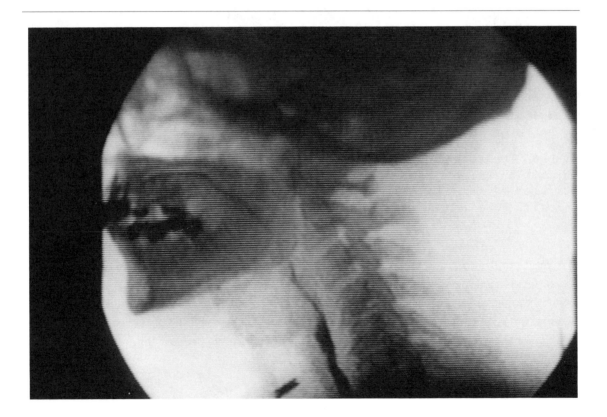

Fig. 6-8 Patient Voluntarily Prolongs Tongue Base Retraction, Laryngeal Elevation, Laryngeal Vestibular Closure, and PES Opening during a Mendelsohn Maneuver

must be taken into consideration when evaluating the efficacy of using these strategies with patients. For example, the airway protective maneuvers such as the supraglottic swallow or the Mendelsohn maneuver may not be realistic with patients who are unable to hold their breath beyond a few seconds or in patients who are unable to coordinate breathing with swallowing (Martin et al., 1992; Selley, Flack, Ellis, & Brooks, 1989b).

Assistive Devices

Palatal Augmentation Prosthesis

Palatal appliances have been used with dysphagic patients who suffer from surgical ablation or neuromuscular impairment of oral structures (Logemann, Sisson, & Wheeler, 1980; Logemann et al., 1989b; Wheeler, Logemann, & Rosen, 1980). The principal role of the palatal appliance is to drop the palatal vault to enhance tongue-to-palate contact (Logemann, 1983). If the soft palate is involved, the prosthesis may be posteriorly extended. Speech production and resonance may also be enhanced. Besides improving the oral aspects of deglutition, case studies have shown that the palatal prosthesis can potentially improve the pharyngeal components of swallow, such as swallow efficiency, duration of tongue contact to the pharyngeal wall, and pharyngeal transit time (Logemann et al., 1989b). The contour of the palatal appliance should be individualized, based on the nature of the patient's structural and functional impairment. Clinical experience shows that the patient must be motivated to tolerate and adapt to the prosthesis during speech and swallowing and will require training regarding optimum oral bolus positioning and compensatory tongue placements for articulation.

CONCLUSION

Compensatory swallowing strategies are typically used in combination with one another and with sensory and cognitive stimulation. The selection of strategies must be based on objective scrutiny of the patient's swallowing impairment(s) and on their proven use during visualization or pressure diagnostic testing. We are beginning to obtain data that support the effectiveness of controlling bolus characteristics, posture, and biofeedback management techniques. We also observe improvement in the functional swallowing ability of our dysphagic patients during our treatment regimes. However, there are several troubling issues that we must consider in our future treatment planning.

There is little empirical evidence to support the treatment efficacy of sensory stimulation or physiotherapeutic exercises as they relate specifically to the treatment of dysphagic patients. Further, we do not understand how sensory or motor pathways may be fatigued by our current therapy methods. Therefore, we must begin to objectify our treatment techniques by quantification of outcome. There are several ways to accomplish this end that are being tested in clinical laboratories. Visual biomechanical evaluation of alterations, particularly improvements in temporal swallowing dynamics and oropharyngeal pressures in relation to bolus movement, are two such objective methods (Dengel et al., 1991; Logemann et al, 1989a; Logemann & McConnel, 1991). Although these types of analyses are time-consuming, documentation of functional swallowing changes in response to specific therapy techniques will clarify the effectiveness of our treatment strategies on durational measures of swallow components (i.e., transit times, laryngeal closure duration, pharyngoesophageal opening), pressure generation, and bolus velocity (Logemann & McConnel, 1991). Quantification of reductions in oral and pharyngeal residue, as well as aspiration, could show objective improvements in swallow efficiency throughout the course of therapy (Hamlet et al., 1989, 1992; Humphreys et al., 1987). Improvements in oral, pharyngeal, laryngeal, and esophageal muscle strength could be confirmed with electromyographic studies (Bryant, 1991; Palmer et al., 1992).

Swallowing clinicians who do not have access to such sophisticated techniques should attempt to quantify clinical outcomes, such as

- decreases in pharyngeal swallow delay time
- increases in the frequency of spontaneous swallows
- advancements to oral feedings
- upgrades in food or liquid textures
- reductions in the degree of required supervision
- improved nutritional status
- decreases in the time required to eat a meal safely (Martin, 1987; Martin et al., 1992)

Corroborative studies with physical and occupational therapists are warranted to improve our understanding and quantification of facilitatory and inhibitory physiotherapeutic and sensory stimulation techniques. The swallowing clinician must become a clinical researcher whose practices are directed toward optimal patient outcomes and validation of dysphagia treatment methods.

REFERENCES

Adnerhill, I., Ekberg, O., & Groher, M.E. (1989). Determining normal bolus size for thin liquids. *Dysphagia, 4,* 1–3.

Aki, B.F., & Blakely, W. (1974). Late assessment of results of cricopharyngeal myotomy for cervical dysphagia. *American Journal of Surgery, 128,* 818–822.

Ardran, G.M., & Kemp, F.H. (1952). The protection of the laryngeal airway during swallowing. *British Journal of Radiology, 25,* 406–416.

Ardran, G.M., & Kemp, F.H. (1967). The mechanism of the larynx. II. The epiglottis and closure of the larynx. *British Journal of Radiology, 40,* 372–389.

Bastian, R.W. (1991). Videoendoscopic evaluation of patients with dysphagia: An adjunct to the modified barium swallow. *Otolaryngology Head and Neck Surgery, 104,* 339–350.

Blakely, W., Garety, E., & Smith, D. (1968). Section of the cricopharyngeus muscle for dysphagia. *Archives of Surgery, 96,* 745–762.

Brown, G.E., Nordloh, S., & Donowitz, A.J. (1992). Systematic desensitization of oral hypersensitivity in a patient with a closed head injury. *Dysphagia, 7,* 138–141.

Bryant, M. (1991). Biofeedback in the treatment of a selected dysphagic patient. *Dysphagia, 6,* 140–144.

Butcher, R.B. (1982). Treatment of chronic aspiration as complication of cerebrovascular accident. *Laryngoscope, 92,* 681–685.

Caruso, A.J., Stanhope, S.J., & McGuire, D.A. (1989). A new technique for acquiring three-dimensional orofacial nonspeech movements. *Dysphagia, 4,* 127–132.

Clark, G. (1920). Deglutition apnoea. *Journal of Physiology, London, 54,* 59.

Curran, J. (1990). Overview of geriatric nutrition. *Dysphagia, 5,* 72–76.

Curran, J., & Groher, M. (1990). Development and dissemination of an aspiration risk reduction diet. *Dysphagia, 5,* 6–12.

Dantes, R.O., Kern, M.K., Massey, B.T., Dodds, W.J., Kahrilas, P.J., Brasseur, J.G., Look, I.J., & Lang, I.M. (1990). Effect of swallowed bolus variables on oral and pharyngeal phases of swallowing. *American Journal of Physiology, 258,* G675–G681.

Dengel, G., Robbins, J., & Rosenbeck, J.C. (1991). Image processing in swallowing and speech research. *Dysphagia, 6,* 30–39.

Doty, R. (1968). Neural organization of deglutition. In C.F. Code (Ed.), *Handbook of Physiology*: Sec. 6. Alimentary canal: Vol. 4, Motility (pp. 1861–1902). Washington, D.C.: American Physiologic Society.

Doty, R., Richmond, W., & Storey, A. (1967). Effect of medullary lesions on coordination of deglutition. *Experimental Neurology, 17,* 91–106.

Dworkin, J.P., & Nadal, J.C. (1991). Nonsurgical treatment of drooling in a patient with closed head injury and severe dysarthria. *Dysphagia, 6,* 40–49.

Hamlet, S., Muz, J., Patterson, R., & Jones, L.A. (1989). Pharyngeal transit time: Assessment with videofluoroscopic and scintigraphic techniques. *Dysphagia, 4,* 4–7.

Hamlet, S., Muz, R., Farris, R., Kumpuris, T., & Jones, L. (1992). Scintigraphic quantification of pharyngeal retention following deglutition. *Dysphagia, 7,* 12–16.

Hotaling, D.L. (1990). Adapting the mealtime environment: Setting the stage for eating. *Dysphagia, 5,* 77–83.

Hukuhara, T., & Okada, H. (1956). Effects of deglutition upon spike discharges of neurons in the respiratory center. *Japanese Journal of Physiology, 6,* 162–166.

Humphreys, B., Mathog, R., Rosen, R., Miller, P., Muz, J., & Nelson, R. (1987). Videofluoroscopic and scintigraphic analysis of dysphagia in the head and neck cancer patient. *Laryngoscope, 97,* 25–32.

Jacob, P., Kahrilas, P., Logemann, J., Shah, V., & Ha, T. (1989). Upper esophageal sphincter opening and modulation during swallowing. *Gastroenterology, 97,* 1469–1478.

Kahrilas, P.J., Logemann, J.A., Krugler, C., & Flanagan, E. (1991). Volitional augmentation of upper esophageal sphincter opening during swallowing. *American Journal of Physiology, 260 (Gastrointestinal Liver Physiology, 23)*: 6450–6456.

Kandel, E.R. (1985). Nerve cells and behavior. In E.R. Kandel and J.H. Schwartz (Eds.), *Principles of neural science* (2nd ed.) (p. 21). New York: Elsevier Science Publishing Co.

Kennedy, J., & Kent, R. (1985). Anatomy and physiology of deglutition and related functions. *Seminars in Speech and Language, 6,* 257–272.

Langmore, S.E., Schatz, K., & Olsen, N. (1988). Fiberoptic endoscopic examination of swallowing safety: A new procedure. *Dysphagia, 2,* 216–219.

Lazzara, G., Lazarus, C., & Logemann, J. (1986). Impact of thermal stimulation on the triggering of the swallow reflex. *Dysphagia, 1,* 73–77.

Linden, P. (1989). Videofluoroscopy in the rehabilitation of swallowing dysfunction. *Dysphagia, 3,* 189–191.

Linden-Castelli, P. (1991). Treatment for adult dysphagia. *Seminars in Speech and Language, 12,* 255–261.

Lof, G., & Robbins, J. (1990). Test–retest variability in normal swallowing. *Dysphagia, 4,* 236–242.

Logemann, J.A. (1983). *Evaluation and treatment of swallowing disorders.* San Diego: College Hill Press.

Logemann, J.A. (1986). *Manual for the videofluorographic study of swallowing.* San Diego: College Hill Press.

Logemann, J.A. (1988). Swallowing physiology and pathophysiology. *Otolaryngolic Clinics of North America, 21,* 613–616.

Logemann, J.A. (1990). Normal swallowing and the effects of oral cancer on normal deglutition. *Head and Neck Cancer, II,* 324–326.

Logemann, J.A., & Kahrilas, P.J. (1990). Relearning to swallow post CVA: Application of maneuvers and indirect biofeedback. A case study. *Neurology, 40,* 1136–1138.

Logemann, J.A., Kahrilas, P.J., Begelman, J., Dodds, W.J., & Pauloski, B.R. (1989a). Interactive computer program for biomechanical analysis of videoradiographic studies of swallowing. *American Journal of Roentgenology, 153,* 277–280.

Logemann, J.A., Kahrilas, P.J., Cheng, J., Pauloski, B.R., Gibbons, P.J., Rademaker, F.W., & Lin, S. (1992a). Closure mechanisms of the laryngeal vestibule during swallow. *American Journal of Physiology, 262,* G388–G344.

Logemann, J.A., Kahrilas, P.J., Hurst, P., Davis, J., & Krugler, C. (1989b). Effects of intraoral prosthetics on swallowing in patients with oral cancer. *Dysphagia, 4,* 118–120.

Logemann, J.A., Kahrilas, P.J., Kobara, M., & Vakil, B. (1989c). The benefit of head rotation on pharyngoesophageal dysphagia. *Archieves of Physical Medicine and Rehabilitation, 70,* 767–771.

Logemann, J.A., & McConnel, F.M.S. (1991). *Cancer control screen project in head and neck cancer rehabilitation, subproject one: Three P01-CA40 007.* Evanston, IL: Northwestern University.

Logemann, J.A., Sisson, G., & Wheeler, R. (1980). The team approach to rehabilitation of surgically treated oral cancer patients. *Proceedings of the National Forum on Cancer Rehabilitation* (pp. 222–227). Williamsburg, VA.

Mansson, I., & Sandberg, N. (1975). Oropharyngeal sensitivity and elicitation of swallowing in man. *Acta Otolaryngologica, 79,* 140–145.

Martin, B.J.W. (1987). Researching, developing, and marketing a comprehensive swallowing program in a health care setting. Gaylord, MI: Northern Speech Services.

Martin, B.J.M. (1991). *The influence of deglutition on respiration.* Doctoral dissertation, Northwestern University, Evanston, IL.

Martin, B.J.M., & Corlew, M.M. (1990). The incidence of communication disorders in dysphagic patients. *Journal of Speech and Hearing Disorders, 55,* 28–32.

Martin, B.J.M., Corlew, M.M., Kirmani, N., & Olson, D. (in press). The association of swallowing dysfunction and aspiration pneumonia. *Dysphagia, 9.*

Martin, B.J.M, Logemann, J.A., Shaker, R., & Dodds, W.J. (1993). Normal laryngeal valving patterns during three breath hold maneuvers: A pilot investigation. *Dysphagia, 8* (1) 11–20.

Martin, B.J.M., Nitschke, T., Schleicher, M., Chachere, K., & Dodds, W.J. (1992). *Frequency of swallowing in adults.* Paper presented at the First Inaugural Dysphagia Research Society, Milwaukee, WI.

McConnel, F.M.S. (1988). Analysis of pressure generation and bolus transit during pharyngeal swallowing. *Laryngoscope, 98,* 71–78.

McConnel, F.M.S., Cerenko, D., & Mendelsohn, M.S. (1988). Manofluorographic analysis of swallowing. *Otolaryngologic Clinics of North America, 21,* 625–637.

McConnel, F.M.S., Mendelsohn, M.S., & Logemann, J.A. (1987). Manofluorography of deglutition after supraglottic laryngectomy. *Head and Neck Surgery, 9,* 142–150.

Miller, A.J. (1982). Deglutition. *Physiological Review, 62,* 129–184.

Mirro, J.F., & Patey, C. (1991). Developing a dysphagia dietary program. *Seminars in Speech and Language: Swallowing Disorders,* 218–227.

Nishino, T., Yonezawa, T., & Honda, Y. (1985). Effects of swallowing on the pattern of continuous respiration in human adults. *American Review of Respiratory Disease, 132,* 1219–1222.

Palmer, J.B., Rudin, N.J., Lara, G., & Crompton, A.W. (1992). Coordination of mastication and swallowing. *Dysphagia, 7,* 187–200.

Perlman, A.L., Grayhack, J.P., & Booth, B.M. (1992). The relationship of vallecular residue to oral involvement, reduced hyoid elevation, and epiglottic function. *Journal of Speech and Hearing Research, 35,* 734–741.

Perlman, A.L., Luschei, E.S., & Du Mond, C.E. (1989). Electrical activity in the superior pharyngeal constrictor muscle during reflexive and non-reflexive tasks. *Journal of Speech and Hearing Research, 32,* 749–754.

Pommerenke, W. (1928). A study of the sensory areas eliciting the swallow reflex. *American Journal of Physiology, 84,* 36–41.

Ramsey, G.H., Watson, J.S., Gramiak, R., & Weinberg, S.A. (1955). Cinefluorographic analysis of the mechanism of swallowing. *Radiology, 64,* 498–518.

Rosenbeck, J.C., Robbins, J., Fishback, B., & Levine, R. (1991). Effects of thermal application on dysphagia after stroke. *Journal of Speech and Hearing Research, 34,* 1257–1267.

Selley, W.G., Flack, F.C., Ellis, R.E., & Brooks, W.A. (1989a). Respiratory patterns associated with swallowing: Part 1. The normal adult pattern and changes with age. *Age and Ageing, 18,* 168–172.

Selley, W.G., Flack, F.C., Ellis, R.E., & Brooks, W.A. (1989b). Respiratory patterns associated with swallowing: Part 2. Neurologically impaired dysphagic patients. *Age and Ageing, 18,* 173–176.

Shawker, T., Sonies, B., Hall, T., & Baum, B.J. (1984a). Ultrasound analysis of tongue, hyoid, and larynx activity during swallowing. *Investigative Radiology, 19,* 82–86.

Shawker, T., Sonies, B., & Stone, M. (1984b). Sonography of speech and swallowing. In R. Sander & M. Hill (Eds.), *Ultrasound Annual* (pp. 237–260). New York: Raven Press.

Smith, J., Wolkove, N., Colacone, A., & Kreisman, H. (1989). Coordination of eating, drinking and breathing in adults. *Chest, 96,* 578–582.

Sonies, B. (1991). Instrumental procedures for dysphagia diagnosis. In B. Sonies (Ed.), *Seminars in Speech and Language: Swallaowing Disorders, 12,* 185–199.

Sonies, B.C., Ship, J.A., & Baum, B.J. (1989). Relationship between saliva production and oropharyngeal swallow in healthy, different-aged adults. *Dysphagia, 4,* 85–89.

Storey, A.T. (1976). Interactions of alimentary and upper respiratory tract reflexes. In B. Sessle and A. Hannam (Eds.), *Mastication and swallowing: Biological and clinical correlates* (pp. 22–36). Toronto: University of Toronto Press.

Sumi,. T. (1963). The activity of brain-stem respiratory neurons and spinal respiratory motoneurons during swallowing. *Journal of Neurophysiology, 26,* 466–477.

Tracy, J.F., Logemann, J.A., Kahrilas, P.J., Jacob, P., Kobara, M., & Krugler, C. (1989). Preliminary observations on the effects of age on oropharyngeal deglutition. *Dysphagia, 4,* 90–94.

Umphred, D.A., & McCormack, G.L. (1985). Classification of common facilitory and inhibitory treatment techniques. In D.A. Umphred (Ed.), *Neurological rehabilitation* (Vol. 3). St. Louis: CV Mosby. Veis, S., Logemann

J., & Kahrilas, P. (1989). *Pattern of closure of the laryngeal vestibule in normal deglutition.* Paper presented at the annual meeting of the Amer

can Speech-Language-Hearing Association, Boston. Wein, B., Bockler, R., & Klajman, S. (1991). Temporal reconstruct on of sonographic imaging of disturbed tongue movements. *Dysphagia, 6,* 135–139. Wheeler, R., Logem

nn, J.A., & Rosen, M. (1980). Maxillary reshaping prostheses: Effectiveness in improving speech and swallowing o post-surgical oral cancer patients. *Journal of Pros

thetic Dentistry, 43,* 313–319.

Wilson, S., Thach, B., Brouillette, R., & Abu-Osba, Y. (1981). Coordination of breathing and swallowing in human infants. *Journal of Applied Physiology, 50,* 851–858.

◆ CHAPTER 7 ◆

Treatment of Feeding and Swallowing Disorders in Children: An Overview

Judy Michels Jelm

Specific treatment goals for the child diagnosed with dysphagia are based on the results of a comprehensive clinical assessment of oral motor, oral sensory, respiratory-phonatory status, posture, muscle tone, positioning, and cognition and language levels. Often, the results of radiographic studies such as videofluoroscopy and ultrasound can further assist in the delineation of appropriate treatment goals. The clinical and radiographic assessments of feeding and swallowing in infants and children have been discussed in Chapters 4 and 5.

In formulating a feeding and swallowing program, it is important to consider whether the feeding problem is congenital or acquired and to delineate goals that are compatible with the child's developmental age (Christensen, 1989). If the dysphagia is acquired and development was previously normal, the child may present with remnants of previously existing skills which can be built on in treatment. Feeding and swallowing rehabilitation is different in children with congenital neurogenic dysphagia because new skills and modifications of existing abnormal patterns must be learned by an impaired nervous system (Christensen, 1989).

This chapter discusses indirect management strategies for daily mealtime feeding such as

- positioning and postural changes
- modifications of food consistency, texture, temperature, and taste
- equipment adaptations

Direct management techniques to facilitate jaw, lip, cheek, and tongue stability and mobility and to facilitate swallowing are also presented. Regardless of the treatment approach, it is important to remember that parental/caregiver involvement is essential to ensure the successful carryover of rehabilitation strategies.

POSTURAL TECHNIQUES

Proper positioning and handling of a child during mealtime is an essential part of the treatment program. Positioning may reduce the impact of limiting reflexive movement patterns of the body and helps provide a central base of stability for oral-motor, oral-pharyngeal, respiratory, and sensory-motor functioning (Alexander, 1987).

The optimal body position to facilitate organized and coordinated oral-motor activity in a child usually consists of the following (Alexander, 1987):

- neck elongation with neutral head flexion
- symmetric and stable shoulder girdle depression with scapulohumeral dissociation
- symmetric trunk elongation
- neutral positioning of a stable and symmetric pelvis
- hip stability with neutral abduction and rotation
- symmetric stable positioning of the feet flat on a surface

Many children assume compensatory postures during feeding to control their head and neck position, to compensate for limiting tone and movement patterns, to compensate for respiratory difficulties, and to protect their airway from aspiration (Morris & Klein, 1987). These compensatory postures may include head or neck hyperextension, head turning, shoulder elevation, desiring to be fed in prone or supine, and leaning forward, backward, or to a particular side.

The position in which a child is most frequently fed may not be the feeding position that is recommended. Any changes in position should be done gradually and with caution. For example, if the position of a child who has favored head or neck hyperextension during feeding is suddenly changed to a different alignment, the child's system may, in fact, be compromised and the chance for aspiration increased rather than decreased (Beecher, 1992). Therefore, it is important to be aware of the positive or negative changes in function that may result from a change in positioning.

It is also important to approach oral-motor treatment from a total body perspective. For example, if an infant or child is in a sitting position, a single weightshift through gentle handling may provide the stimulation necessary for symmetrical control of the pelvis, allow for improved respiratory patterns, and facilitate improved oral-motor movements for feeding. When a change in position is indicated for a child who demonstrates concurrent orthopedic or tonal problems, consultation with the physical and/or occupational therapists is always advisable.

Recommended postural changes may include head rotation to the weaker side to improve unilateral pharyngeal or laryngeal weakness (Logemann, 1990) or slight head and neck extension to improve airway alignment. Either slight to moderate head and neck hyperextension or slight chin tuck combined with a change in food consistency may assist with increased bolus movement within the oral cavity.

A postural change of any kind should be explained fully to the feeder and to the child, when appropriate. Postural changes with children almost always directly affect how a parent/caregiver holds the child or positions themselves when feeding the child. During feeding, it is important that both the child and the caregiver be comfortable. Wedges, pillows, and adaptive equipment can assist in this area.

SENSORY STIMULATION: MODIFYING FOOD CONSISTENCY, TEXTURE, TEMPERATURE, AND TASTE

The specific sensory properties of a food may facilitate more normal oral movements during feeding (Morris & Klein, 1987). Therefore, a change in food consistency, texture, temperature, and/ or taste may be recommended to improve the child's ability to bite, chew, and propel a bolus through the oropharynx. Any modifications to the sensory components of food should be done only after careful consideration of the effects. For example, a soft solid that is easier to bite may, at the same time, be more difficult to chew because chewing skills require increased and coordinated tongue movement patterns that are not required for biting.

Thicker, heavier foods provide more tactile and proprioceptive cues, thereby facilitating more active jaw, tongue, and cheek/lip movements in chewing and bolus formation. Also, because thicker foods move more slowly through the oral and pharyngeal cavities and do not splash into the airway, they may be effective for children with problems protecting the airway. In contrast, change to a thinner consistency is recommended for children who demonstrate, for example, reduced pharyngeal peristalsis.

Moistened solids may be used for children who have difficulty controlling foods that crumble during chewing (e.g., cookies) because of movement dysfunctions of the lips/cheeks, tongue, or jaw. When a solid is moistened, it tends to "clump," thus assisting with bolus formation.

It is helpful to measure the amount of the thickening agent that is added to the food to alter its consistency. It is also helpful to describe for the parent/caregiver and child the texture of the liquid or solid (e.g., smooth, thin, thick, dry, moist, lumpy, easily chewable, hard to chew, grainy, mushy, crunchy, or any combination of these). Specific measurements and descriptions will assist the parent/caregiver in selecting other foods that have similar sensory components, and will aid in the carryover of goals to different settings. They also allow feeding progress to be measured as additives are decreased and textures modified.

Changing the temperature of the bolus has been effective for children with delayed initiation of the pharyngeal swallow. When the bolus temperature is changed from tepid to chilled, the child appears to demonstrate greater awareness within the oral cavity, thus facilitating a swallow that is initiated with greater speed (Morris & Klein, 1987). Similarly, Wolf and Glass (1991) successfully used chilled formula during nutritive sucking to speed the initiation of the pharyngeal swallow with infants in whom it was delayed.

The clinician should be aware that cold temperature and light touch frequently increase tone adversely in those children who demonstrate hypertonicity or hypersensitivity. Very warm or very cold foods may also be uncomfortable for the child with dental problems. Changes in consistency and temperature should be introduced gradually, and their effects should be monitored carefully, because individual response to sensory change varies depending on the child's overall state. Attempt at all times to provide the infant or child with foods that are pleasurable. If an infant or child perceives food as noxious, refusal to eat, gagging, spitting, or vomiting may occur (Morris & Klein, 1987).

Modifying the taste of the foods may be beneficial for children who demonstrate hyper- or hyposensitivity. Enhancing the flavor of a food may result in better bolus formation and quicker bolus propulsion within the oral cavity as the child becomes increasingly aware that food is presented within the oral cavity. If the child's diet allows, moderate amounts of salt, pepper, spices, and imitation flavored extracts (nonalcoholic) are useful for enhancing flavor. Before initiating a feeding program, it is always advisable to obtain information about the child's specific dietary requirements (e.g., caloric restrictions, food allergies).

EQUIPMENT ADAPTATIONS

The types and sizes of utensils used in feeding may affect oral-motor functioning. Careful selection of adaptive feeding equipment may assist with bolus formation and may reduce the speed of "flow" of the bolus. For example, slow-flow nipples are useful for infants who demonstrate difficulty controlling the quick flow of thin liquids because of poorly organized tongue movement. Different shapes, sizes, and textures of nipples should be tried to see which allow for more active tongue and jaw activity during bottle drinking (Alexander, 1987).

When children are learning to cup-drink, different sizes and shapes of cups may facilitate a desired response. A cut-out cup may facilitate improved tongue positioning for some children and is most beneficial for those children who require slight head/neck flexion. A cup with a sipper seal may improve independent lip-cheek function. However, sipper seals may also facilitate an unwanted extension–retraction movement pattern of the tongue and should be introduced with caution. When possible, children should be introduced to a variety of cups that meet their oral motor needs.

Adaptive equipment also includes small bowled spoons, different shaped spoons, and latex-covered spoons. Maroon spoons are made from a hard, smooth plastic and are available in two bowl sizes. Use the small, shallow-bowled spoon for infants and young children. The larger spoon is appropriate for children who demonstrate active upper lip activity; they can independently use their upper lip to remove food from the spoon. The maroon spoon, or a latex-covered spoon should be used for a child with a tonic bite. Avoid touching the teeth or side gums of a child with a tonic bite, because hypersensitivity to touch in this oral area appears to be associated with tonic biting.

Much of the adaptive feeding equipment is commercially available through specialty catalogs. Appendix 7-A lists several companies that offer this equipment. It is also useful to scan the baby product section of the local food and department stores for new products.

ORAL-MOTOR STRATEGIES

In many children, oral preparatory dysfunctions are a key problem. Effective treatment techniques initially focus on improving jaw, lip-cheek, and tongue stability and movement (Jelm, 1987); then, when appropriate, oral-motor feeding strategies are introduced. Many of these treatment strategies have evolved from the principles of Bobath and Bobath (1964) and are taught as part of the Pediatric 8-Week Neuro-Developmental Treatment Course.

Jaw Stability and Mobility

Jaw stability and related ability to grade jaw movement are of prime importance. The jaw is the "foundation of support" (Jelm, 1988) for the tongue and lip-cheek mobility. If the jaw is not stable in a child or adult, active and coordinated tongue and lip-cheek mobility is greatly compromised and cannot be expected. It is difficult to suck, bite, chew, and swallow while experiencing unstable, ungraded jaw movement.

With this premise as a basis for treatment, close attention should always be given to the jaw and all aspects of its movement capabilities during the feeding process. If jaw movement is compromised, providing external jaw stability through oral control is often beneficial.

Oral control may be used during bottle feeding, spoon feeding, cup drinking, biting, and chewing. Two basic hand positions that provide oral control have been described (Mueller, 1975).

Oral Control from the Side

The feeder may either hold the child or the child may be positioned in a small seat at the side of the feeder. The feeder uses one hand to hold the utensil or food item; the other arm is positioned around the back of the child with the hand positioned as follows (Fig. 7-1).

1. The fleshy bottom portion of the midfinger is placed horizontally across the tongue base under the jaw. The midfinger movement is vertical and dynamic allowing for improved jaw grading ability. Its dynamic movement may also provide for improved tongue mobility because it is placed horizontally across the tongue base. If the midfinger is placed posteriorly to the tongue base, it may cause tongue retraction as it moves against the hyoid. If placed too far forward, this finger would be positioned on the anterior portion of the mandible, usually providing very little support to the jaw. Providing jaw support forward should only be used if finger position on the tongue base interferes with tongue shaping.

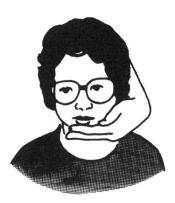

Fig. 7-1 Oral Control from the Side: Classic Position

2. The index finger is placed horizontally across the indentation below the lower lip. Index finger movement is inward and dynamic, allowing for improved lower lip stability and mobility. Movement of the midfinger under the chin and movement of the index finger occur independently of each other.
3. The thumb is tucked away to not cause interference such as pushing on the cheek and forcing the child's face to one side.

Oral Control from the Front

In this technique, the feeder is positioned in front of the child, face to face (Fig. 7-2). Although this position provides less control than the side position, it is effective in providing improved jaw stability, jaw grading, and tongue mobility.

1. The index finger is crooked under the child's chin, the front portion at the tongue base.
2. The thumb, in a vertical position, is placed at the indentation beneath the lower lip. Inward pressure of the thumb facilitates lower lip stability.

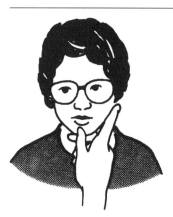

Fig. 7-2 Oral Control from the Front: Classic Position

Several other hand position variations are available, depending on the need and age of each individual child. These may include

1. using the little finger with dynamic pressure at the base of the tongue under the mandible for infants and small children. Very young children who do not display significant tongue shaping difficulties may only need slight pressure under the mandible
2. using only the thumb or midfinger at the base of the tongue
3. above positions (1 and 2) with the addition of index finger support at the lips to increase lip mobility and closure

When providing any form of oral control, the feeder should always monitor the pressure provided to the jaw and lips and cheeks. The goal of oral control is for the child to gain internal graded jaw movement ability. Therefore, varying the pressure throughout the feeding session can help assess whether the child is gaining this internal control with less external control provided directly by the feeder.

Also, the feeder should not constantly move the external hand support on and off the face of the child during the feeding process. Providing continuous sensory and tactile input is much more effective.

Lip-Cheek Stability and Mobility

Although oral control by itself may assist lip and cheek mobility, many children need added support at the cheeks. This improves and assists with propulsion of the food bolus from the front of the mouth to the back of the mouth in readiness for the swallow.

It is difficult to separate lip and cheek function, as both structures generally are co-active. Adequate bilateral lip movements assist with both liquid and solid intake. Bilateral cheek movement also assists with intraoral pressure and bolus formation. If cheek musculature is weak, bolus formation may be affected as both solids and liquids may be lost in the lateral sulci. Without adequate cheek musculature involvement, intraoral pressure variations will also be affected. A useful technique is to face the child, place hand(s) directly on the child's cheeks, and provide direct and dynamic inward pressure to the cheeks as the bolus is being moved within the oral cavity. This inward pressure should be varied from the corners of the mouth toward the molar area in a wave-like fashion in response to bolus formation and movement. The addition of oral control with the thumb(s) under the child's jaw, together with external support to the lips-cheeks is also advisable.

Tongue Stability and Mobility

When providing oral control, stability is added at the tongue base, allowing the tongue to move actively and independently from the jaw. As the jaw remains stable, improved active mobility of other tongue movement patterns may be facilitated including

- tongue extension

- tongue retraction
- tongue elevation (elevation may be facilitated in posterior, anterior, mid, and lateral tongue areas)

Oral control may be combined with variations of spoon feeding, cup drinking, biting, and chewing. Equipment (spoon, cup, nipple) and equipment placement within the mouth can be critical. For example, if pureed food is introduced with a spoon that has a bowl that is too deep for the child, all oral-motor movement activity will be adversely affected. The lips will not be able to clean the food off the spoon, and atypical tongue movements may develop to compensate for inadequate lip and cheek activity. However, if that same pureed food is fed using the appropriate-sized spoon and placed directly on the tongue with slight downward pressure, lateral tongue elevation (tongue cupping) can be facilitated.

Tongue cupping can also be facilitated by slowly sweeping forward with slight downward pressure on the central portion of the tongue toward the lips, using a gloved finger or a swab with a handle. The maroon spoons, as described earlier, are useful also for this goal.

Cup placement affects oral motor movement control. Placement of the cup should be on the lower lip toward the lip corners for those children requiring greater jaw stability. As a child gains internal jaw grading ability, cup placement should be moved forward on the lower lip. Oral control may be used to provide external jaw stability if necessary.

Facilitating the Swallow

Before the introduction of any foods, it is critical to determine whether a pharyngeal swallow is present. If the swallow is absent, food and liquid should not be used during the program. Rather, treatment should focus on enhancing sensory and motor skills within the oral cavity, without using food (Morris, 1989).

Certain strategies that appear to be effective with adults, such as thermal stimulation, may not be beneficial for children younger than 5 years of age. Most children who are younger than 5 years of age are too young to cooperate fully and to consistently follow the directions needed to use compensatory strategies. Using chilled nipples, formula, and foods, as described previously, may assist with stimulation of a swallow in children younger than 5 years.

Increasing the strength, duration, and rhythm of the suckle pattern may result in the initiation of a swallow (Morris, 1989). The clinician may facilitate a suckle by using a finger to stroke the tongue rhythmically in a downward and forward motion. Once a suckling pattern at a rate of approximately one per second emerges, water, juice, or small amounts of pureed fruits may be added to the stroking finger. Larger amounts of food are gradually added to the rhythmic tongue movements of the suckle by stroking with drops of liquid on a swab or from a medicine dropper or syringe. Later, when the child is able to handle larger amounts from a spoon, the rhythm can be sustained by tipping the front of the spoon downward and touching the tongue with rhythmic contact on the tip (Morris, 1989).

TREATING THE INFANT OR CHILD WHO IS RECEIVING NONORAL FEEDINGS

Many infants and children receive their nutrition through nonoral tube feedings such as a gastrostomy, jejunostomy, or nasogastric tube. Abnormal tone and movement patterns, respiratory problems, swallowing disorders, gastroesophageal reflux, or abnormal responses to oral stimulation have been noted in infants who are fed nonorally (Morris, 1989). Children who are fed nonorally may display a regression of oral motor skills, which includes

- loss of suck/swallow coordination
- immature lingual and mandibular movement patterns
- oral hypersensitivity (Monahan, Shapiro, & Fox, 1988)

In addition to the physical problems, other related factors may interfere with the development of the feeding process. Infants may not always experience bonding with the parent/caregiver, and children may not experience the social interaction that usually occurs during mealtime. Poor social interactive skills during feeding may result in poor caloric intake, vomiting, or aversion to food (Ramsey & Zelazo, 1988). Thus, these children may have a variety of problems, as a result of or in addition to the nonoral feeding, that contribute to the feeding and swallowing problems. Therefore, these children require special consideration.

Before working with an infant or child who is fed nonorally, it is essential to determine if he or she has always been fed by alternate means, has received oral feeding in the past, or is receiving a combination of the two types of feeding. It is also important to determine the reasons for the tube feedings and whether there is a history of or risk for aspiration. Those children who are fed nonorally as a result of respiratory dysfunction interfering with the breathing-swallowing coordination demonstrate increased risk for aspiration and must be carefully monitored by the treatment team.

Some children who are fed nonorally may demonstrate specific oral-motor problem areas such as poor mandibular strength, poor mandibular grading, poor lingual-buccal function, or lingual movement pattern dysfunction. Generally, postural changes combined with oral-motor techniques are beneficial for children who demonstrate motor-based oral problems.

Other children who are fed nonorally may demonstrate a disorganized oral sensory system. An oral stimulation treatment program that incorporates all sensory systems (oral, gustatory, tactile, visual, auditory, vestibular, and proprioceptive) should begin as quickly as possible. Oral stimulation activities may include using a gloved finger to rub the child's gums and to provide sensory input to the tongue. Also, allow the child to mouth and suck on toys, pacifiers, or fingers. Oral exploration and play should be a daily experience. Attempt at all times to make facial and oral sensory input a pleasurable and joyful experience. Many oral movement patterns and strengthening of these movement patterns of the tongue, lips-cheeks, and jaw can be facilitated with oral facilitation play.

Oral facilitation techniques to facilitate improved oral sensory experiences in preparation for possible oral feeding at a later date should be considered. For example, wrap gauze around food items and allow the child to maneuver the item in the oral cavity while the clinician holds the other end of the gauze strip. This allows the child to discover and experiment with a variety of tastes and temperatures without the possibility of swallowing a solid. Biting and chewing (jaw grading) can also be facilitated in this manner as the thickness and texture of the food is altered. Exhibit 7-1 provides general treatment guidelines for the child who is fed nonorally.

Exhibit 7-1 General Treatment Guidelines for the Child Who is Fed Nonorally

1. If it is recommended that a child take nothing by mouth (NPO), introduce oral stimulation techniques within and around the oral cavity as soon as possible. Oral play should be provided many times during the day for short periods of time.

2. Soothing music used in conjunction with oral stimulation techniques often calms an agitated child (Morris & Klein, 1987).

3. Provide oral stimulation during mealtime (tube feedings) to build an association between oral sensation and hunger satiation.

4. During oral play allow the child to become aware of age appropriate feeding equipment such as the nipple, spoon, and cup.

5. Oral motor sensory stimulation often results in increased salivation. Working with the child in antigravity positions such as prone or sidelying will reduce aspiration risks for children who display difficulty handling their own saliva.

6. When oral feeding is recommended by the child's physician, begin by introducing very small tastes, perhaps on the end of the spoon or on a finger—feeding equipment that is already familiar to the child. If the child resists, stop and try again later. If the child is upset, oral motor coordination may break down and the risk for aspiration will increase.

7. Use the recommended position for the child. Be constantly aware of any position changes that the child may make indicating distress.

8. The transfer from tube feeding to oral feeding occurs very slowly. When the child has become accustomed to a taste, slowly introduce greater volumes (for example, 3 to 5 very small spoonfuls, with food placed at the end of the spoon).

9. Present the oral feeding immediately before the tube feeding in order that the association between reduced hunger and oral feeding continues.

10. When the child is able to orally feed these small volumes consistently, with no aversive response, a videofluoroscopic or ultrasound swallow study may be recommended. This may indicate whether the child should continue to increase oral feeding volume and reduce tube feeding volume.

11. As caloric and nutrient intake by mouth increases, intake through the tube will be reduced. Consultation with a nutritionist to set up an individual feeding plan that incorporates both tube feeding and oral feeding is recommended to ensure that the child receives the proper nutritional diet.

12. Developmentally appropriate feeding skills such as drinking, biting, and chewing are introduced with appropriate liquid and/or solid consistency and texture as the child progresses.

SUMMARY

This chapter has discussed indirect management strategies for daily mealtime feeding such as positioning, modification of the sensory properties of the food, and equipment adaptations. Direct management strategies to facilitate jaw, lip, cheek, and tongue stability and mobility and to facilitate swallowing have been reviewed. Also, some suggestions for treating children who are fed nonorally have been presented. The development, implementation, and carryover of a successful feeding and swallowing program is dependent on careful observation, analysis, and treatment of the whole child. Therefore, involvement of the entire team, which may include the parent/caregiver, physician, nurse, dietitian, speech-language pathologist, occupational therapist, physical therapist, and teacher, is an important component of the program.

REFERENCES

Alexander, R. (1987). Oral-motor treatment for infants and young children with cerebral palsy. *Seminars in Speech and Language, 8* (1), 87–100.

Beecher, R. (1992). Pediatric Feeding Problems (from Inside Out). Paper presented at the 5th Annual Neuro-Developmental Treatment Association Conference. Denver, CO.

Bobath, K., & Bobath, B. (1964). The facilitation of normal postural reactions and movements in the treatment of cerebral palsy. *Physiotherapy, 50,* 246–262.

Christensen, J.R. (1989). Developmental approach to pediatric neurogenic dysphagia. *Dysphagia, 3,* 131–134.

Jelm, J.M. (1987). Assessment and Treatment of Oral Motor Dysfunction. Workshop sponsored by Continuing Education Resource, Inc. Anaheim, CA.

Jelm, J.M. (1988). Assessment and Treatment of Oral Motor Dysfunction. Workshop sponsored by Continuing Education Resource, Inc. Columbus, OH.

Logemann, J.A. (1990). Infant Swallowing. Miniseminar presented at the Annual Convention of the Illinois Speech Language Hearing Association. Chicago, IL.

Monahan, P., Shapiro, B., & Fox, C. (1988). Effect of tube feeding on oral function. *Developmental Medicine and Child Neurology, 57* (Suppl), 7.

Morris, S.E. (1989). Development of oral-motor skills in the neurologically impaired child receiving non-oral feedings. *Dysphagia, 3,* 135–154.

Morris, S.E., & Klein, M.D. (1987). *Pre-feeding skills: A comprehensive resource for feeding development.* Tucson, AZ: Therapy Skill Builders.

Mueller, H. (1975). Feeding. In N.R. Finnie (Ed.), *Handling the young cerebral palsied child at home* (2nd ed., pp. 113–132). New York: E.P. Dutton.

Ramsay, M., & Zelazo, P. (1988). Food refusal in failure-to-thrive infants: Nasogastric feeding combined with interactive behavioral treatment. *Journal of Pediatric Psychology, 13,* 329–347.

Wolf, L.S., & Glass, R.P. (1991). *Feeding and swallowing disorders in infancy: Assessment and management.* Tucson, AZ: Therapy Skill Builders.

APPENDIX 7-A

Companies Offering Commercially Available Feeding Equipment

Ansa Bottle Company, Inc.
1107 W. Shawnee
Muskogee, OK 74401

The Equipment Shop
P.O. Box 33
Bedford, MA 01730

Evenflo Products Company
771 N. Freedom Street
Ravena, OH 44266

Gerber Products Company
445 State Street
Fremont, MI 49412

Johnson and Johnson Baby Products
Skillman, NJ 08558

La Leche League International
9616 Minneapolis Avenue
Franklin Park, IL 60131

Mead Johnson Company
Nutritional Division
Evansville, IN 60014

Mealtimes
c/o New Visions
Route 1 Box 175-S
Faber, VA 22938

Playtex
P.O. Box 728
Paramus, NJ 07652

Roylan Medical Products
P.O. Box 555
Menominee Falls, WI 53051

Fred Sammons, Inc.
Pediatric Catalog
P.O. Box 32
Brookfield, IL 60513

Therapy Skill Builders
3830 E. Bellevue
P.O. Box 42050-C91
Tucson, AZ 85733

◆ CHAPTER 8 ◆

Developing Quality Assurance Monitors for Dysphagia: Continuous Quality Improvement

Anita S. Halper and Leora R. Cherney

A comprehensive dysphagia program involves the evaluation and treatment of the dysphagia as well as procedures for evaluating and monitoring the effectiveness of the program. The purpose of this chapter is to review the current guidelines prescribed by the Joint Commission on the Accreditation of Health Care Organizations (JCAHO) for monitoring and evaluating the quality and appropriateness of patient care and to present sample monitors for the management of dysphagic patients.

The JCAHO is a private, not-for-profit organization dedicated to improving the quality of patient care in organized health care settings. Quality assurance is the planned and systematic means of evaluating and monitoring patient care quality. Patient care quality has been defined as

> The degree to which patient care services increase the probability of desired patient outcomes and reduce the probability of undesired outcomes, given the current state of knowledge. (Patterson, 1990)

Patient care quality is a continuous rather than a static process, because the probability of desired patient outcomes always can be improved. In addition, treatment procedures and the hospital systems that support patient care can also be improved.

Source: Reprinted with permission from *Seminars in Speech and Language*, Vol. 12, No. 3, pp. 228–235. Copyright © 1991 by Thieme Medical Publishers, Inc. 381 Park Avenue South, New York, NY 10016. All rights reserved.

The JCAHO is in the process of redesigning its standards to focus on *continuous quality improvement* rather than quality assurance. The philosophy of continuous quality improvement does not conflict with quality assurance but is broader, more comprehensive, and hospital-wide (Schiff et al., 1990). It cuts across all departments within an organization and emphasizes the interdependence of one department or team on the other. The concept of customer is expanded to focus not only on the receiver of services (patient) but also on the provider (Re and Krousel-Wood, 1990). For example, when speech-language pathologists utilize the services of the Scheduling Department, they become a consumer of services of that department.

MONITORING AND EVALUATION PROCESS

JCAHO currently has a ten-step process for monitoring and evaluating the quality and appropriateness of patient care. These steps also reflect the continuous quality improvement philosophy (Schiff, 1990). They are as follows (Patterson and Schyve, 1989; Schiff, 1990):

1. *Identify and assign responsibilities:* The appropriate person (e.g., director of a clinical department, chair medical staff committee) defines and designates the responsibilities of others in performing monitoring and evaluation activities.
2. *Delineate scope of care:* The scope of care for a clinical service involves all major clinical functions related to comprehensive patient management (evaluation, treatment, discharge planning, and follow-up). The types of patients, their diagnoses, and the types of treatment provided (e.g., individual, group) also should be included.
3. *Identify important aspects of care:* The monitoring and evaluation process should focus on the important aspects of care. The activities chosen should impact on a large number of patients, occur frequently, and/or previously have produced problems. Priority also is given to those activities that if incorrectly provided, put patients at risk.
4. *Identify indicators:* Indicators are succinct, objective statements that define specific aspects of patient care. Indicators must be measurable and well defined. An indicator may relate to the structure, process, or outcome of care (Patterson and Schyve, 1989). Structures refer to factors such as resources, equipment, and qualifications and numbers of staff. Processes refer to functions carried out by staff such as assessment, treatment planning, and management of complications. Outcome refers to the short- and long-term results of management procedures, as well as any complications.
5. *Establish thresholds for evaluation:* These thresholds are established for each indicator and serve as the level at which further evaluation is required.
6. *Collect and organize data:* The sample size, frequency of data collection and analysis, method of review, and responsible staff are determined.
7. *Evaluate care:* If the results show that the indicator does not meet the preestablished thresholds, the staff should evaluate the data to determine whether a problem is present.

8. *Take action to improve care:* If it has been determined that a problem exists, appropriate corrective action should be taken.
9. *Assess actions:* There should be continued monitoring and evaluation to assess the effectiveness of the corrective action.
10. *Communicate information:* Pertinent information should be communicated to appropriate individuals within the department and the facility.

MONITORING AND EVALUATING THE MANAGEMENT OF DYSPHAGIA

For the purposes of developing clinical monitors for dysphagia, we have found it useful to divide patients into two groups. One group consists of those patients who receive most of their nutrition via alternative feeding methods; any oral intake is provided only by the speech-language pathologist. Therefore, a departmental clinical monitor is used. In contrast, an interdisciplinary monitor is required for the other group. This group of patients receives oral intake under the supervision of both the nursing staff and the speech-language pathologist. Sample monitors for both of these groups are presented. In addition, a departmental monitor that focuses on treatment planning and outcome is included.

Departmental Clinical Monitors

Monitor for Dysphagic Patients Receiving Oral Intake Only from the Speech-Language Pathologist

The Department of Communicative Disorders' Quality Assurance Committee became aware of the need to monitor and evaluate the care provided to high-risk dysphagic patients in the early stages of treatment who were receiving oral intake only from the speech-language pathologist. The primary nutritional needs of these patients were being met by an alternative feeding method. Table 8-1 illustrates this monitor.

The important aspect of care identified was treatment of dysphagic patients. Two indicators, an outcome indicator and a process indicator, were defined:

- *Indicator 1:* This measure of outcome states that the high-risk dysphagic patients will not develop any related complications such as aspiration pneumonia.
- *Indicator 2:* The Dysphagia Treatment Plan is used to document information collected immediately prior to and during each treatment session. In addition, any subsequent modifications to the treatment plan are noted. The items on the plan were carefully selected to ensure patient safety and to help a clinician make decisions regarding the dysphagia program.

The Dysphagia Treatment Plan in high-risk dysplagic patients, which is used to document daily and weekly progress, is shown in Exhibit 8-1. The information obtained prior to a treatment session

Table 8-1. Important Aspect of Care: Dysphagia Treatment for Patients Receiving Oral Intake Only from the Speech-Language Pathologist

Indicators	Threshold for Evaluation
1. High-risk dysphagic patients (receiving oral intake only from the speech-language pathologist) do not develop any complications	100%
2. The information on the dysphagia treatment plan is complete	100%
Sample size: All high-risk dysphagic patients	
Frequency of data collection: Daily	
Frequency of data evaluation: Monthly	
Method of review: Dysphagia treatment plan	
Responsible party: The speech-language pathologist or clinical supervisor treating the patient completes the Dysphagia Treatment Plan form and the Department Quality Assurance Committee analyzes the data	

helps the speech-language pathologist identify signs of possible aspiration that might have occurred since the last treatment session. This information is typically obtained from the medical record or from verbal reports of nursing staff or physicians and includes the following: the presence of a fever, changes in the amount and quality of secretions, changes in the frequency of suctioning required, and changes in the frequency of the coughing. Other pertinent information that might affect the decision to orally feed the patient on a particular day should also be documented (e.g., presence of urinary tract infection, seizures, and changes in medical status, respiratory rate, or medications). It is important to consider such information, since the presence of fever, for example, may result from a urinary tract infection rather than any factor related to oral intake.

Based on the above information, the clinician decides whether to change the patient's treatment. For example, the patient who has a fever may be kept NPO (no oral feeding) for that day. A patient whose performance during and after oral intake has been stable for several days without signs of difficulty may have their food consistency upgraded, the amount given per mouthful increased, or the length of treatment sessions increased.

It is unrealistic to administer a videofluoroscopic examination during every treatment session. Therefore, the speech-language pathologist must rely on clinical observations as indicators of possible aspiration. The dysphagia treatment plan includes those clinical indicators that are relevant to most high-risk dysphagic patients. The patient's level of responsiveness, including the presence of

Exhibit 8-1 Rehabilitation Institute of Chicago Department of Communicative Disorders—High-Risk Dysphagic Patients

Pt. Name _____
RIC # _____
Clinician _____

SOURCE KEY: P = Physician   N = Nursing   M = Medical Record   N/P = Not Pertinent   N/A = Not Available

Information Obtained Prior to Treatment:	*Monday* Date ___ Source ___	*Tuesday* Date ___ Source ___	*Wednesday* Date ___ Source ___	*Thursday* Date ___ Source ___	*Friday* Date ___ Source ___	*Saturday* Date ___ Source ___				
Does patient have a fever?										
Any change in secretions? (amount/quality)										
Any change in frequency of suctioning?										
Any change in frequency of coughing?										
Other:										
Treatment Approach Changed?										
Information Obtained During Treatment:										
Patient's level of responsiveness										
Frequency of coughing										
How much food was eaten?										
What kind of food?										
Any change in vocal quality following swallowing?										
Any complaints of discomfort/obstruction in throat during swallow?										
How many times patient suctioned during session?										
Was patient suctioned at the end of the session?										
Length of session										
Other										
Treatment Approach to be Changed?										

agitation, distractibility, impulsivity, or other behavioral characteristics that would interfere with the patient's dysphagia program, is noted.

Coughing is a sign of the patient's ability to protect the airway. The number of episodes of coughing within a designated time period is documented initially. Any subsequent increase or decrease in coughing should be noted. In addition, changes in voice quality after swallowing may indicate pooling at the laryngeal level. If the patient complains of discomfort during or after swallowing, it may be a sign of reduced cricopharyngeal functioning. The speech-language pathologist should note the consistency of such complaints and ask the patient to indicate the site of discomfort.

The Dysphagia Treatment Plan also includes the consistency (e.g., thick liquids, pureed) and the amount of food eaten (e.g., number of ounces, teaspoons, calories). The length of each treatment session is indicated so that the amount of each consistency that is swallowed in a given time period can be calculated on a daily basis. For those patients with a tracheostomy tube, the number of times that suctioning was needed during a session is noted. In addition, the speech-language pathologist indicates whether suctioning was given at the end of session. Other pertinent information that affects the current treatment plan is also documented.

Considering all the information obtained during the current session and in previous sessions, the speech-language pathologist makes a decision regarding changes to be implemented. This may include upgrading food consistency or allowing the patient to be fed by the nursing staff and/or family.

The threshold for evaluation has been set at 100 percent for both indicators. It is important that all items on the Dysphagia Treatment Plan be completed to ensure that the speech-language pathologist does not overlook essential information. The monitor is used with all dysphagic patients receiving oral intake only from the speech-language pathologist. The daily data, collected by the speech-language pathology staff, are analyzed monthly by the Department's Quality Assurance Committee. Corrective actions are taken when appropriate.

Treatment Planning and Outcome Monitor

A second departmental need was to evaluate the appropriateness of the treatment plans developed for all dysphagic patients and the outcome effectiveness. Therefore, the important aspect of care identified was treatment planning and outcome for all dysphagic patients. Two indicators were delineated (Table 8-2):

- *Indicator 1:* The process indicator that short-term goals for dysphagia are appropriate for the patient is evaluated through a peer review process. If the goals are determined to be appropriate, then Indicator 2 is completed. If the goals are not appropriate, Indicator 2 is not considered because outcome is dependent on the appropriateness of the treatment plan.

- *Indicator 2:* Outcome is measured by the achievement of the appropriate goal.

The threshold for evaluation was set at 100 percent for Indicator 1. It was determined that all goals should be appropriate for patient quality care and corrective action should be taken even if only one goal is inappropriate. On the other hand, Indicator 2 was set at 85 percent because there are justifiable reasons why a goal might not be met (e.g., medical problems, poor attendance to treatment, unexpected behavioral problems).

The sample that is analyzed consists of all dysphagic patients treated during a specific 1-week period every 2 months. The Department's Quality Assurance Committee analyzes the department chart and progress notes. The previous progress note is reviewed for goal appropriateness, while the current progress note is reviewed for outcome. Two members of the Committee observe the patient's treatment session if confirmation of the appropriateness of the goal is needed. Corrective action is taken as indicated.

In our department, long-term outcome is evaluated via another mechanism. The Rehabilitation Institute of Chicago (RIC) (1989) has a functional assessment scale that is used at admission and discharge. The RIC's Program Evaluation and Follow-up staff collect admission and discharge ratings determined by the speech-language pathologist. One of the items relates to functional feeding status, which includes food consistency, degree of supervision, and whether alternative feeding methods are required for nutritional support. The data permit additional assessment of outcome to be made.

Table 8-2 Important Aspect of Care: Dysphagia Treatment Planning and Outcome

Indicators	Threshold for Evaluation
1. Short-term goals for dysphagia are appropriate for the patient	100%
2. Patient achieved appropriate short-term goals for dysphagia	85%
Sample size: All dysphagic patients during a 1-week period of time bimonthly	
Frequency of data collection: Bimonthly	
Frequency of data evaluation: Bimonthly	
Method of review: Communicative Disorders' Department chart, progress notes, and observation of patient if confirmation is needed	
Responsible party: The Department Quality Assurance Committee analyzes the data to determine if the goals are appropriate and met	

Interdisciplinary Clinical Monitor

The development of an interdisciplinary monitor for dysphagia patients being fed and/or supervised by both nursing and speech-language pathology staff required the expertise of both of these disciplines. In particular, the nursing staff provided input regarding selection of indicators that would help determine proper nutritional and fluid intake. Table 8-3 illustrates the interdisciplinary monitor.

First, the important aspect of care identified by both the Nursing and Communicative Disorders departments was defined as effective management of dysphagia by the staff of the respective departments. Five clinical indicators were agreed on. Indicator 1, 3, and 4 are process indicators. Indicator 5 is an outcome indicator and Indicator 2 is both.

- *Indicator 1:* The patient's nutrition/fluid program, which includes the consistency of the diet, prescribed fluids, and the necessary compensatory techniques, is documented completely in the Nursing Patient Care Summary. These instructions are essential for managing the nutritional aspects of a dysphagic patient's care. Documentation in the Patient Care Summary is essential to ensure that these are communicated to the appropriate nursing staff.

- *Indicator 2:* Fluid intake and urine output are measured and calorie counts documented daily in the medical record. Therefore, the speech-language pathologist is also responsible for collecting any fluid and caloric intake data. In addition, patients are weighed two times a week. These measures help determine whether the patient is receiving adequate nutrition and fluid. Thus, this indicator measures both the process and the outcome of adequate nutrition and fluid intake.

- *Indicator 3:* Prescribed compensatory techniques, as determined by the speech-language pathologist, are described in the Patient Care Summary. Correct implementation of these techniques is determined through observation of the patient at each meal for a 24-hour period. These observations are done by the Communicative Disorders Supervisor and/or the Assistant Clinical Director of Nursing on each nursing unit.

- *Indicator 4:* Every 2 weeks the patient's program is reviewed by both Nursing and Communicative Disorders staff and modified accordingly. The modifications are documented in the Patient Care Summary.

- *Indicator 5:* The indicator that the patient does not develop aspiration pneumonia is an important measure of outcome.

Thresholds for evaluation were set at 100 percent because of the importance of ensuring that every patient was being fed safely, receiving adequate nutrition, and not developing aspiration pneumonia. Data from a sample size of ten patients on each of the nursing units are collected and analyzed on a quarterly basis. Appropriate corrective actions are taken as indicated by the Communicative Disorder's Supervisor and the Assistant Clinical Director of Nursing on each nursing unit.

Table 8-3 Important Aspect of Care: Dysphagia Treatment by the Communicative Disorders and Nursing Staff

Indicators	Thresholds for Evaluation
1. Nutrition/fluid program is listed on Patient Care Summary (program is defined as consistency of diet, prescribed fluids, and necessary compensatory techniques)	100%
2. Data are collected and documented as prescribed, to evaluate nutrition/fluid intake including intake/output, calorie counts, and weights twice a week	100%
3. Prescribed compensatory techniques listed in the Patient Care Summary are implemented as prescribed	100%
4. Documentation indicates assessment and evaluation of nutrition/fluid program at least every 2 weeks	100%
5. Patient does not develop complications of aspiration pneumonia during treatment	100%

Sample size: 10 patients per nursing unit quarterly

Frequency of data collection: Quarterly

Frequency of data analysis: Quarterly

Method of review: Nursing Patient Care Summary, medical record, and observation of patient at each meal for a 24-hour period

Responsible party: Communicative Disorders Supervisor and Assistant Clinical Director of Nursing on each nursing unit

SUMMARY

The purpose of this article is to highlight the importance of developing a method of systematically evaluating and monitoring the effectiveness of a dysphagia program. Specific departmental and interdisciplinary monitors that conform to the standards of the JCAHO have been presented. These monitors include both process and outcome indicators. They are specific to our rehabilitation facility and may need to be modified for other facilities.

ACKNOWLEDGMENT

We thank Jean Deddo, B.S.N., R.N., Manager, Quality Assurance and Utilization Review, Rehabilitation Institute of Chicago, for her thoughtful comments on an earlier draft of this chapter.

REFERENCES

Patterson, C.H. (1990). *From quality assurance to quality improvement.* Keynote Address presented at a Continuing Education Course, A Collaborative Approach: Linking Quality Assurance, Program Evaluation and Follow-up and Utilization Review in Rehabilitation, Rehabilitation Institute of Chicago, Chicago, Illinois.

Patterson, C.H., & Schyve, P.M. (1989). Quality assurance. In B. England, R.M. Glass, & C.H. Patterson (Eds.), *Quality rehabilitation: Results-oriented patient care* (pp. 39–51). Chicago: American Hospital Publishing.

Re, R.N., & Krousel-Wood, M.A. (1990). How to use continuous quality improvement theory and statistic quality control tools in a multispecialty clinic. *Quality Review Bulletin: Journal of Quality Assurance, 16,* 391–397.

Rehabilitation Institute of Chicago (1989). *RIC—FAS II: Rehabilitation Institute of Chicago Functional Assessment Scale.* Chicago: Rehabilitation Institute of Chicago.

Schiff, L.P. (1990). Quality improvement and the JCAHO. In *Conference Proceedings of the Second Annual Quest for Quality and Productivity in Health Services* (pp. 186–191). Chicago, IL: Society for Health Systems and Healthcare Information Management Systems Society.

Schiff, L.P., Smith, M., Feather, H., McPhail, V., Fainter, J., & Buchanan, E.D. (1990). The opportunities of quality improvement compared to the traditional quality assurance program. In *Conference Proceedings of the Second Annual Quest for Quality and Productivity in Health Services* (pp. 173–177). Chicago, IL: Society for Health Systems and Healthcare Information Management Systems Society.

RIC Clinical Evaluation of Dysphagia (CED)

Leora Reiff Cherney, Ph.D., CCC-SP
Carol Addy Cantieri, M.A., CCC-SP
Jean Jones Pannell, MA., CCC-SP

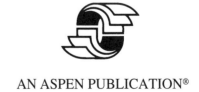

AN ASPEN PUBLICATION®

Clinical Evaluation of Dysphagia
Face Sheet

Patient: _____ Date: _____

Case #: _____ Therapist: _____

Overall diagnosis: _____
_____

Dysphagia severity: _____
_____

Suggestions for feeding: _____
_____
_____
_____
_____
_____
_____
_____

Recommended diet: _____
_____
_____

Precautions: _____
_____
_____
_____
_____
_____
_____
_____
_____

Name: _____

Case #: _____

Date: _____

Evaluation of Prefeeding Skills

Medical/Nutritional Status _____

_____

_____

Respiratory Status _____

History of Aspiration _____

Tracheostomy _____ yes _____ no   Type _____   Size _____

   Position of Cuff _____ Inflated _____ Partially Inflated _____ Deflated

   Suctioning Required _____ yes _____ no   Frequency _____

   Other Relevant Information_____

Level of Responsiveness _____

Behavioral Characteristics _____

Current Feeding Method   Oral _____   Alternate _____

   Intake Amount _____   Frequency of Intake _____

   Other _____

Positioning

Habitual _____

Interfering Patterns _____

Trial/Optimal Position _____

_____

Observations of Oral, Pharyngeal, and Laryngeal Function

Lips _____

Tongue _____

Mandible _____

Name: _____

Date: _____

Dentition _____

Phonation _____

Articulation _____

Hypernasality _____   Hyponasality _____

Cough (involuntary and volitional) _____

Gag Reflex _____

Voluntary Swallow _____

Other Observations _____

Response to Stimulation

_____

_____

_____

_____

_____

Recommendations

_____ Swallowing Evaluation Deferred: Patient NPO

_____ Clinical Evaluation of Swallowing

_____ Videofluoroscopy

_____ ENT

_____ Other _____

_____

Goals:

_____

_____

_____

_____

_____

_____

_____

Patient/Family Counseling:

_____

_____

_____

THIN LIQUIDS | THICK LIQUIDS | PUREED | GROUND SOLIDS | CHOPPED SOLIDS | REGULAR SOLIDS

Name: _____

Case #: _____

Date: _____

General Impressions: _____
_____

I. *ORAL STAGE*

A. *Lips*

1. Protrusion

	Spoon	Cup	Straw

_____ Initiates protrusion

_____ Maintains protrusion

2. Closure

_____ Initiates Closure for Retrieval from Utensil

_____ Maintains Closure for Retrieval from Utensil

_____ Maintains Closure throughout Oral Stage

_____ Leakage _____

3. Interpretation of Lip Function

_____ Adequate

_____ Adequate but Reduced

_____ Interferes with Function

_____ Nonfunctional

Problems due to

_____ ↓ ↑ Tone

_____ ↓ Sensation

_____ ↓ Strength

_____ ↓ Range of Motion

_____ ↓ Rate

_____ Inaccurate Direction

_____ Other_____

B. *Tongue*

1. Bolus Formation and Transport

_____ Adequate

_____ Adequate but Reduced

_____ Interferes with Function

_____ Nonfunctional

_____ Pumping Action of Tongue

_____ Tongue Thrust

2. Food Remaining in Mouth

_____ None

_____ Left Side

_____ Right Side

_____ Anterior

_____ Roof of Mouth

_____ Midline of Tongue

_____ On Lips

THIN LIQUIDS | THICK LIQUIDS | PUREED | GROUND SOLIDS | CHOPPED SOLIDS | REGULAR SOLIDS

B. *Tongue* (cont.)

   3. Cough Reflex before Swallow

      _____ Yes

      _____ No

   4. Interpretation of Tongue Function

      _____ Adequate

      _____ Adequate but Reduced Function

      _____ Interferes with Function

      _____ Nonfunctional

      Problems due to

         _____ ↓ ↑ Tone

         _____ ↓ Elevation

         _____ ↓ Range of Motion Within Oral Cavity

         _____ ↓ External Range of Motion

         _____ ↓ Rate

         _____ ↓ Sensation

         _____ ↓ Strength

         _____ Inaccurate Direction

         _____ Other

C. *Mandible/Muscles of Mastication*

   1. Chewing

      _____ Rotary

      _____ Vertical

      _____ Absent

   2. Interpretation of Mandibular Function

      _____ Adequate

      _____ Adequate but Reduced Function

      _____ Interferes with Function

      _____ Nonfunctional

      Problems due to

         _____ ↓ ↑ Tone

         _____ Abnormal Reflexes (list)

         _____

         _____ ↓ Strength

         _____ ↓ Range of Motion

         _____ ↓ Rate

         _____ Dentition _____

         _____ Occlusion

         _____ Other

THIN LIQUIDS
THICK LIQUIDS
PUREED
GROUND SOLIDS
CHOPPED SOLIDS
REGULAR SOLIDS

Name: _____
Date: _____

D. *Summary*

Overall Oral Phase

_____ Adequate

_____ Adequate but Reduced Function

_____ Interferes with Function

_____ Nonfunctional

Problems due to _____

_____

Additional Comments: (Medical or behavioral status that *compensates* or *interferes* with performance)

_____

_____

_____

II. *PHARYNGEAL PHASE*

Gag Reflex   present   diminished   absent

Volitional Cough   present   diminished   absent

_____ Cough Reflex before Swallow

_____ Nasal Regurgitation

_____ Elevation of Hyoid and Thyroid Cartilage Observed

_____ Delayed Pharyngeal Swallow   _____ seconds

_____ Repeated Swallows   Average number per bolus _____

_____ Complaints of Discomfort/Obstruction in Throat during

Swallow (specify location) _____

_____ Cough Reflex during Swallow

_____ Cough Reflex after Swallow

_____ Vocal Quality after Swallow

Describe _____

_____ Excessive Copious Secretions

_____ No Problems Exhibited

THIN LIQUIDS | THICK LIQUIDS | PUREED | GROUND SOLIDS | CHOPPED SOLIDS | REGULAR SOLIDS

Name: _____
Date: _____

A. *Summary*
   Overall Pharyngeal Phase
   _____ Adequate
   _____ Adequate but Reduced Function
   _____ Interferes with Function
   _____ Nonfunctional
   Problems due to_____
   _____
   _____
   _____

   Patient Appears Able/Unable to Protect Airway
   Additional Comments (e.g., medical or behavioral status that *compensates*
   or *interferes* with performance)_____
   _____
   _____
   _____

III. *ADDITIONAL TEST RESULTS*
     Videofluoroscopy Test Results/Recommendations
     _____
     _____
     _____
     _____
     _____
     _____
     _____

     ENT Test Results _____
     _____
     _____
     Other _____

IV. *OVERALL FUNCTIONAL SEVERITY LEVEL AND INTERPRETATION OF UNDERYLING*
    NEUROMUSCULAR CHARACTERISTICS
    _____
    _____
    _____
    _____
    _____

Clinical Management of Dysphagia in Adults and Children
Copyright © 1994 by Aspen Publishers, Inc.
CED-7

CED-EDUCATIONAL MATERIALS

Schematic Drawing of Structures and Areas
Involved in the Swallowing Process

Soft Palate

Pharynx

Epiglottis

Upper esophageal sphincter

Esophagus

Tongue

Larynx

Vocal cords

Trachea

KATZ

To Lungs

To Stomach

Name: _____

Date: _____

Normal Feeding Process

1. Food taken into mouth
2. Food chewed
3. Food moved to back of mouth
4. Swallow is initiated as follows:

   a) soft palate rises to block the nasal passageway
   b) muscles in the pharynx move the food downward (process of peristalsis)
   c) vocal cords in the larynx close to protect the airway
   d) upper esophageal sphincter opens, allowing food to pass into the esophagus
   e) upper esophageal sphincter closes to prevent regurgitation of food back into the pharynx and possibly the airway
   f) food continues through digestive tract by action of peristalsis

Malfunction of one or more of any of the following structures/processes can cause feeding difficulties.

Problem areas are circled and explained below:

LIPS   SOFT PALATE

TEETH   PHARYNX

MUSCLES OF CHEEK AND/OR   VOCAL CORDS/OTHER
  JAW (FOR CHEWING)   LARYNGEAL MUSCLES

TONGUE   UPPER ESOPHAGEAL SPHINCTER

INITIATION OF SWALLOW   ESOPHAGUS

Description of Problems:

_____
_____
_____
_____
_____
_____
_____
_____
_____
_____
_____

Name: _____

Date: _____

Suggestions for Feeding:

1. Not ready to be fed. _____

2. Ready to be fed by the speech-language pathologist only._____

3. Ready to be fed by nursing staff or family members familiar with the specific feeding program.

_____

4. Ready to self-feed with close supervision by trained staff and/or trained family members.

_____

5. Ready to self-feed with occasional supervision. _____

6. Independent self-feeding. _____

Recommended Diet:

Food consistencies to be used:_____

_____

Food consistencies to be avoided: _____

_____

Feeding Techniques to Use:

Positioning: _____

_____

_____

Presentation/placement of food: _____

_____

_____

Other: _____

_____

_____

_____

If you have any further questions, please contact: _____

RIC Clinical Evaluation of Dysphagia: Pediatrics (CED—Pediatrics)

Wendy S. Perlin, MA, CCC-SLP
Maureen M. Boner, MS, CCC-SLP

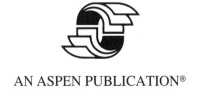

AN ASPEN PUBLICATION®

Name: _____

Case #: _____

Date of Birth: _____ Age: ____

Date of Evaluation: _____

Parent/Caregiver Questionnaire

Parent/Caregiver Interviewed: _____

1. In what position and seating system do you usually feed your child?

2. Are any special utensils or equipment used? (Please list)

3. Do you use any special feeding techniques? (Please list)

4. What are your child's likes and dislikes (foods, textures, temperatures)? (Please list)

5. What foods or beverages are difficult for your child to eat or drink? How so?

6. How long does it usually take to feed your child an average meal?

7. How much food does your child usually eat in one meal? (Describe an average meal.)

8. Do you supplement your child's oral diet in any way?

9. Has your child had any unusual problems with eating (e.g., reflux, food or liquid leaking from the nose)?

10. Was the introduction of solid foods difficult? How so?

11. Is there any history of allergies, asthma, or dietary restrictions?

12. Who usually feeds the child?

Name: _____

Case #: _____

Date of Birth: _____   Age: _____

Date of Evaluation: _____

Preassessment

BEHAVIOR
Age-appropriate:
Reduced attention:
Impulsivity:
Fatigue:
Agitation:
Manipulative behaviors (please list):

Other:

POSITIONING
Habitual feeding position:

Trial/optimal feeding position:

INTERFERING PATTERNS
Overall tone:
Primitive reflexes:

Abnormal patterns/posturing:

RESPIRATION
Within normal limits:
Raspy:
Labored:
Mouth-breather:
Other:

Clavicular:
Thoracic:
Abdominal:
Asthma:
Stridor:

FEEDING EQUIPMENT
Utensils (type and grip):

Cup (type):   Straw:

Bottle/nipple type:

Other:

TRACHEOSTOMY TUBE
Present:
Type:
Cuff:
One-way valve:
Frequency of suctioning:
Corking schedule:

Size:
Fenestrated:
Type:

ORAL INTAKE
Formula type:
Type of food eaten:
Amount per oral feeding:
      Liquid: _____ Solid: _____
Frequency of oral feedings:
      Liquid: _____ Solid: _____
Duration of average feeding:
History of intolerance:
      Type of food/liquid:
Other:

ALTERNATE FEEDING
Method of alternate feeding:
Supplemental formula:
Intake amount:
Time after last feeding:
Other:

MEDICAL CONTRAINDICATIONS
Fever: G-E reflux:
Tracheoesophageal fistula:
Tracheomalacia:
Other:

Name: _____ Date of Birth: _____

Case #: _____ Date of Evaluation: _____ Age: _____

	Sensation		Symmetry	Tone		Related Features	Elicited Movements					
	Sensation Right	Left	Symmetry	Tone Right	Left	Circle as appropriate or comment	Elicited Individual or Repetitive	RANGE	RATE	STRENGTH	COORDI-NATION	Comments
FACE						Dysmorphic features:		L/R	L/R	L/R		
LIPS						Tremor / Retraction / Dysmorphic features:	Retraction / Protraction / Compression					
TONGUE						Tremor / Retraction / Bunched / Fasciculations / Short frenulum / Atrophy / Dysmorphic features:	Lateralization / Cheek pushes / Circular range of motion / Protrusion / Elevation outside lips / Elevation to hard palate / Depression					
DENTITION AND JAW						Good hygiene / Prosthesis / Missing teeth / Dental bite / Bruxism	Jaw opening					
PALATE						Arch: High / Flat / Normal Cleft: Type:						
VELO-PHARYNX						Tonsils: / Uvula:	Elevation on phonation / Nasality: WNL ___ Hypernasal ___ Hyponasal ___	L R	L R	L R		
PHARYNX/LARYNX	Gag ___ Hyper ___ Hypo ___						VOCAL QUALITY Clear ___ Wet ___ Laryngeal elevation on dry swallow: Present ___ Absent ___ Reduced ___					

KEY: N = Normal/Symmetric; R = Reduced; E = Excessive; I = Irregular; D = Deviant/Asymmetric

Clinical Management of Dysphagia in Adults and Children
Copyright © 1994 by Aspen Publishers, Inc.
CED-Pediatrics-3

The Pediatric Scale

Name: _____

Case #: _____

Date of Birth: _____ Age: ____

Date of Evaluation: _____

Age in Months:	0–3	4–6	7–9			10–12		
Reflexes								
Rooting								
Babkin								
Palmomental								
Transverse tongue								
Bite								
Gag								
Startle								
Grasp								
ATNR								
Face								
Varied facial expressions								
Recognition of bottle/utensil								
Anticipation of food/liquid								
	Bottle	Bottle	Bottle	Cup	Spoon/Fork	Bottle	Cup	Spoon/Fork
Lips								
Approximation								
Active lip closure								
Active lip movement								
Active pull on nipple								
Maintain lip closure								
Liquid/food lost								
Remove food from utensil								
Tongue								
Cupped configuration								
Protrusion on swallow								
Lateralization								
Ability to form bolus								
Good posterior movement of food/liquid								
Ability to clean lips								
Dentition/Mandible								
Wide excursion								
Good jaw control								
Ability to bite off cookie								
Stability by biting on cup								
Vertical chew								
Rotary chew								
Ability to initiate and maintain chewing								
Coordination								
Active suck								
Active suckle								
# Suck(le)s before breath	2–3	20	20+			20+		

Key: Present (P) Still present some of the time (P*) Emerging skill (EM) Absent (A) Not applicable

Name: _____

Case #: _____

Date of Birth: _____ Age: _____

Date of Evaluation: _____

Age in Months:	13–18			19–24			24+	
Reflexes								
Rooting								
Babkin								
Palmomental								
Transverse tongue								
Bite								
Gag								
Startle								
Grasp								
ATNR								
Face								
Varied facial expressions								
Recognition of bottle/utensil								
Anticipation of food/liquid								
	Bottle	Cup	Spoon/Fork	Bottle	Cup	Spoon/Fork	Cup	Spoon/Fork
Lips								
Approximation								
Active lip closure								
Active lip movement								
Active pull on nipple								
Maintain lip closure								
Liquid/food lost								
Remove food from utensil								
Tongue								
Cupped configuration								
Protrusion on swallow								
Lateralization								
Ability to form bolus								
Good posterior movement of food/liquid								
Ability to clean lips								
Dentition/Mandible								
Wide excursion								
Good jaw control								
Ability to bite off cookie								
Stability by biting on cup								
Vertical chew								
Rotary chew								
Ability to initiate and maintain chewing								
Coordination								
Active suck								
Active suckle								
# Suck(le)s before breath	20+			20+				

Key: Present (P)   Still present some of the time (P*)   Emerging skill (EM)   Absent (A)   Not applicable

Name: _____   Date of Birth: _____ Age: ____

Case #: _____   Date of Evaluation: _____

Summary of Feeding and Swallowing Patterns

General Impressions: _____

Interaction: _____

Interfering Patterns and Behaviors: _____

	Thin Liquid	Thick Liquid	Pureed Food	Ground Food	Chopped Food	Regular Food	Comments
LIPS							
Lip retraction							
Lip pursing:							
Loss of liquid: (Unilateral: ____ Bilateral: ____)							
Loss of food: (Unilateral: ____ Bilateral: ____)							
Increased drooling: ____							
No Problems Exhibited: ____							
TONGUE							
Residue in oral cavity:							
Pooling:							
Food packed in palate:							
Pocketing (Location: _____):							
Tongue thrust:							
Tongue retraction:							
Oral transit times (No. of sec):							
No Problems Exhibited: ____							
DENTITION/MANDIBLE							
Jaw thrust:							
Tonic bite reflex (Trigger point: _____):							
Jaw clenching:							
Munching/vertical chew:							
Bruxism:							
No Problems Exhibited: ____							
SWALLOWING							
Delayed trigger of pharyngeal swallow (No. of sec):							
Absent trigger of pharyngeal swallow:							
Swallows per bolus (List number):							
Wet vocal quality before the swallow:							
Wet vocal quality after the swallow:							
Cough before swallow:							
Cough during swallow:							
Cough after swallow:							
Reduced laryngeal elevation:							
No Problems Exhibited: ____							

RESULTS

RECOMMENDATIONS

Clinical Management of Dysphagia in Adults and Children

Index